MW01489961

PREDIABETES

The Definitive Guide

to Reversing Diabetes Naturally

Without the Use of Drugs

Discover the Scientifically Proven Method to Reduce Insulin Resistance and Prevent Type 2 Diabetes

Rebeca Smith & Alison Brown

By reading this document, the reader agrees that under no circumstances is the author responsible for any losses, direct or indirect, that are incurred as a result of the use of information contained within this document, including, but not limited to, errors, omissions, or inaccuracies.

Table Of Contents

Introduction

There is a growing epidemic in the United States that affects millions of people across all age groups and races. This epidemic is diabetes or prediabetes and the number of people who have it has tripled over the last three decades. In September 2019, the Behavioral Risk Factor Surveillance System (BRFSS) found that around 100 million people in America have diabetes *or* prediabetes and many do not know they have it. That's 40% of the population, according to Centers for Disease Control and Prevention (CDC). Furthermore, it's estimated that 30% of people who are living with prediabetes are likely to develop Type 2 diabetes, unless they make drastic changes to their lifestyle habits.

A study carried out at the Institute for Alternative Futures in Alexandria, Virginia has concluded that in spite of advances in medicine, diabetes will continue to be a major health concern for many Americans as both Type 1 and Type 2 diabetes is expected to continue to rise by 54% between 2015 and 2030. This will mean more than 54.9 million Americans will be living with this disease. In addition, the study predicts that annual deaths related to diabetes will increase to 38% (385,800).

At present, adults who are living with diabetes have a 50% increased risk of death from *any cause* than those adults who do not have diabetes. Medical and societal costs will also climb to around $622 billion by 2030. Given the growing concern for the alarming rate at which diabetes is increasing, the CDC publishes diabetes statistics every two years to provide an accurate picture of the diabetic epidemic for the country. The study, which was carried out by the main researcher, Rowley WR (2017), has stated that: *"Reducing this burden will require efforts on many fronts—from appropriate medical care to significant health efforts and individual behavior change across the nation...Public awareness is a key first step."* (2017).

Is There a Solution to Diabetes?

Fortunately, numerous research has been carried out over the years that shows Type 2 diabetes and prediabetes can be prevented or reversed without medication. In fact, professionals in the conventional medicine field have acknowledged that Type 2 diabetes can be avoided by maintaining a healthy diet, regular exercise, and becoming better informed about the disease. For many years it has been widely accepted that when someone is 'struck' by a disease there is absolutely no cure and they are doomed. While we're not suggesting that every single person who contracts a disease is guaranteed to be cured, there are a number of diseases which can be reversed or prevented in the first place. Type 2 diabetes is certainly one of them.

The term 'disease' originally comes from old French before it was used in Middle English, and means "lack of ease." So, when the body has a disease, it really means there is 'dis-ease,' or an imbalance.

A patient who isn't educated on the body's intelligence and is desperate for a cure, or at the very least, assistance with their problem, will take heed of the doctor's standard advice. Many will walk away feeling discouraged that they have to live with the disease and resign themselves to the idea of having to depend on drugs for the remainder of their lives. They're hindered to a large degree and identify so strongly with the disease that their bodies deteriorate even further, over time. For example, someone may say, "I am diabetic." The truth is, they are not 'diabetic.' Sure, they may have diabetes but they are not diabetes itself! This way of talking and thinking doesn't allow the person to be in an empowered state of mind where they can begin to take back control of their body by listening to and providing it with what it requires. Actually, disease or dis-ease is a message from the body that there is disharmony and an imbalance that needs to be restored. It isn't a message to say, *You're doomed, like it or not, and if you're lucky you might only lose your limbs or eyesight at some point!*"

Diabetes is a disease that has been deeply ingrained in society as being chronic; once you have it, that's it, accept your fate because you'll have it for life. Fortunately, there have been studies that prove Type 2 diabetes can be reversed. Although there are some studies that conclude diabetes Type 2 can be reversed with lifestyle changes *and* drugs such as metformin, there are other studies which prove it can be reversed *without* the use of prescriptive medication.

Professor Roy Taylor at the University of Newcastle in the United Kingdom, has carried out extensive research into what causes Type 2 diabetes and how it can be reversed. We will discuss the causes of diabetes and prediabetes in chapter one. However, suffice it to say that by using innovative methods, Taylor has discovered that Type 2 diabetes can be reversed to a point where the person doesn't need to take medication. A trial was undertaken called DiRect (Diabetes Remission Clinical Trial), which was headed by Professor Taylor and Professor Mike Lean at Glasgow University. The trial intended to gain a deeper understanding of diabetes by aiming to see if:

1. Type 2 diabetes can be reversed with care and effort; and

2. Whether the long-term effects of treatment is better than using conventional treatment.

The results of the first half of the trial, which were published in 2017, found that people who had Type 2 diabetes within the first six years were able to reverse the disease after following a low-calorie diet programme. The trial also found that nearly nine out of 10 people who had lost a substantial amount of weight (at least 15kg) went into remission with Type 2 diabetes. It's especially promising that the study also discovered that even after a year, almost half of these patients still didn't need to take their diabetes medication yet maintained normal blood glucose levels.

The University of Newcastle has stated that:

"Our work has shown that type 2 diabetes is not inevitably progressive and life-long. By identifying the cause of the condition it has been possible to design appropriate management. We have demonstrated that in many people who have had type 2 diabetes for up to 10 years, major weight loss returns insulin secretion to normal..." (2019).

What Are the Benefits of Reversing Prediabetes?

According to the National Institute of Diabetes and Digestive and Kidney Diseases (NIDDK), people who are screened for prediabetes and treated for it are more likely to:

● Experience a five to seven percent reduction in weight loss due to healthy lifestyle changes. This includes more physical activity, less sick days at work, and reducing their prescription drugs for high cholesterol and high blood pressure.

- Not have to deal with the stress of having Type 2 diabetes.

- Not have to worry about medical costs and travel insurance costs for having Type 2 diabetes.

What Are the Benefits of Reversing Diabetes?

People who have reversed diabetes has discovered:

- Being able to come off their diabetic medication.

- Dramatic weight loss which has helped to normalize their metabolism and stabilize their blood sugar levels.

- Feeling a strong sense of achievement with their health.

- Saving money on their life and travel insurances.

- Higher quality of life.

- Lower risk of developing other health issues, including heart disease.

- Reduction with other health issues including obesity, chronic illness, inflammation, high blood pressure, and cardiovascular disease.

- More conscious of their general health.

- Greater sense of well-being.

In addition to these benefits for the individual, as more people start to reverse or take preventative measures, it reduces overall health costs for the economy. For instance, Virta Health has stated, *"The total economic burden of diagnosed type 2 diabetes alone in the United States is now near $300 billion..."* (Virta Health 2018).

Now that we know there's plenty of evidence that shows Type 2 diabetes and prediabetes can be reversed, it's important to allow yourself to be open to the possibility that you too can go into remission from diabetes.

The first step in your healing journey is to acknowledge that people have reversed the disease and it's possible for you to join the growing number of individuals who have been able to do this without the use of prescription drugs. Next, it's important that you educate yourself as much as possible on diabetes. This ebook aims to be a guide to help you (or someone you know who is living with the disease) to get a strong understanding of diabetes, and how it can be treated. This book isn't just about the theory of diabetes, it's also a practical handbook that will provide you with specific steps you can take to reverse Type 2 diabetes in as little as eight weeks! Don't be fooled because although it can be reversed in just two months, the results can be long-term.

In chapter one, we will get a clear understanding of prediabetes and diabetes, their causes, and whether they are really curable. It's important that we start to change our perception on diabetes and gain a strong understanding that it can be cured. This can be difficult for many people—including doctors and general practitioners—to grasp, due to many years of conditioning by conventional Western medicine. However, in this ebook we will delve deep into how prediabetes is curable as this will help to change your mindset and prepare you for a healthier lifestyle change that is sustainable over the long haul. In chapter two, we will gain an in-depth understanding of the diagnosis and discuss what symptoms you can expect with the onset of the disease. Chapter three will provide you with three effective tips to reduce insulin resistance *naturally*. Remember, you don't have to rely on drugs to manage your diabetes, there are other ways to heal yourself. We will take a look at the ways you can really start to shift your mindset with the disease. By chapter four, it will be time to explore your dietary options and exercise regime; two crucial aspects to recovering from the disease. Also, we will look into managing stress as this plays a vital role in bringing your body back into equilibrium.

To further retrain your mind, we will discuss the new approaches to diabetes in chapter five. We will first need to see how it has been treated in the past and then look at how it's being approached today. In chapter six, you will learn specific ways to start reversing Type 2 diabetes within weeks. Chapter seven will hone in on a specific diet known as the ketogenic diet, which has been clinically proven by Virta. In chapter eight, you will gain a good understanding of meal plans you can adopt that will help you to reverse diabetes in a way that feels right for you. Chapter nine contains plenty of delicious recipes for breakfast, lunch, evening meals, desserts, and snacks that you can choose from. This diet will allow your body to balance itself back to a state of equilibrium and health, however it doesn't mean the recipes are unappetizing—far from it! You will be pleased to know that the saying, "Good medicine tastes bad" doesn't apply here!

In chapter 10 you will learn how to tap into the body's intelligence system. This is essential and probably not spoken about enough. Your body knows what's best for you and even if you've ignored its messages previously, it's not too late to start now. Chapter 11 will examine the importance of living clean; this includes a healthy clean body, mind, and external environment. All of these components are required if you are to build a healthy lifestyle where diabetes or prediabetes have no place. The conclusion will summarize the important topics discussed in this book and you should feel confident and ready to change your life for the better.

While it's not too late to start listening to your body, the earlier you start to make changes, the better! Therefore we urge you to take the actions as suggested in this book, as soon as possible. Please do not just read through the book and then put it down without first having put in 100% effort. Your body is a gift that works extremely hard to look after you, so you can live the best life possible. Even if you are in a great deal of pain at times, pain is a messenger because it is your body's way of letting you know something needs to be addressed. So, now that we're living in a time where we have a better understanding of how to treat diabetes, let's take advantage of it!

Chapter 1: Defining Prediabetes and Its Causes

What is Diabetes?

Many people have heard of diabetes but they haven't heard of prediabetes, even though they may be living with it and not be aware. And, although diabetes is widely known, many people are not truly aware of what exactly it is. Before we define prediabetes let's first gain a deeper understanding of what diabetes is.

The pancreas produces a hormone called insulin which keeps blood sugar levels balanced in the body. If the body doesn't produce adequate insulin then carbohydrates won't be burned up properly and blood sugar levels (glucose) will become too high. This creates diabetes. We all need some glucose as it helps to provide the body with energy. When we consume food and drink glucose is released into the blood. For someone who doesn't have diabetes, the pancreas is able to detect when glucose enters the bloodstream and is able to release a healthy amount of insulin so that the glucose can access the body's cells. When someone has diabetes, this process doesn't occur.

There are two main types of diabetes: Type 1 and Type 2.

Type 1 Diabetes

This type (previously called insulin dependent diabetes) is known to be chronic and irreversible. People tend to develop it before the age of 35 and approximately 10% of people with diabetes are living with Type 1.

Type 1 diabetes occurs when the pancreas is unable to produce insulin whatsoever because the body attacks the cells that produce it. Even though people with Type 1 can still break down food and turn it into glucose, once it enters the bloodstream there isn't any insulin that allows sugar to enter into the cells. This results in high amounts of glucose building up in the bloodstream. The body will do what it can to get rid of high sugar levels in the blood by eliminating it through the kidneys, resulting in frequent urination. Unfortunately, this causes further problems such as feeling very thirsty. Also, since glucose can't access the cells to provide energy, the person will experience fatigue. As a desperate attempt to try and get energy, the body will break down fat to make fuel. This is why people often experience drastic weight loss before they discover they have Type 1 diabetes.

Since someone with Type 1 diabetes doesn't produce any insulin, they need to either inject it into the body at regular intervals to help stabilize blood sugar levels or use a pump. They also need to monitor blood (glucose) levels several times a day to ensure they are not too high or too low with the use of a blood glucose testing device.

When people start to gain adequate levels of insulin they report feeling better, especially as their blood glucose levels decrease. It can't be emphasized enough the serious long-term consequences for someone who has high glucose levels in the blood. For instance, high blood glucose levels can damage a person's eyes, heart, feet, and kidneys. These are often referred to as the "complications of diabetes." It's currently known that Type 1 diabetes can be managed in the long-run.

It's still generally unknown as to why some people get Type 1 diabetes as many researchers cannot currently find a link between Type 1 and diet. According to Diabetes UK, "It just happens." Although there's currently much research that acknowledges Type 2 can be reversed, there are a few studies starting to emerge which suggest even Type 1 diabetes could be cured. However, the studies are few and far between at the time of this book being published. Nevertheless, there is still hope considering that up until recently it was assumed that there was no way to reverse or prevent Type 2 diabetes. Since we know that Type 2 diabetes can be reversed, this book will focus more on this condition.

Type 2 Diabetes

This is also known as non-insulin dependent diabetes and approximately 90% of people who are living with diabetes have Type 2. It's not uncommon for people to develop this over the age of 40 and it's very commonly found in people who are elderly. While Type 2 diabetes does produce some insulin, it isn't enough or the amount the pancreas makes isn't working efficiently. Unlike Type 1, people often find they have problems with excess weight.

With Type 2 diabetes, the body still breaks down carbohydrates once food and drink have been consumed, and turns it into glucose. The pancreas then release insulin. However, since the insulin is unable to work efficiently or not enough is produced, the blood glucose levels continue to increase and therefore even more insulin is released. Over time, in some individuals this can leave the pancreas exhausted and their bodies make even less insulin. This then creates higher glucose levels in the bloodstream and the person ends up feeling extremely tired. Extreme thirst, the need to urinate frequently, getting infections often, and slow healing of bruises are some symptoms. Unfortunately, there's a reason diabetes is often referred to as a "silent killer." Many people don't get symptoms and often people can live with Type 2 for as long as 10 years before it's diagnosed.

It is often said that Type 2 diabetes can be caused by:

- A history of people in the family who have Type 2 diabetes.

- A person being overweight or obese, especially if they are carrying excess weight around the tummy.

- Age. The older a person is, the more likely they are to develop diabetes, according to studies. This is due to long-term unhealthy eating habits and lifestyle choices.

- The body not receiving adequate exercise. A study carried out at the University of Missouri Institute has shown that not undertaking regular physical activity hinders glycemic control (the control of blood sugar levels). This suggests that remaining inactive plays a primary role in the onset of Type 2 diabetes: *"In the study, Thyfault monitored the activity levels and diets of healthy and moderately active young adults. Participants then reduced their physical activity by 50 percent for three days while replicating the diet they consumed when they were active. Continuous glucose monitors worn by the subjects during the period of inactivity revealed significantly increased levels of PPG. Spikes in blood glucose after meals can indicate increased risks for type 2 diabetes and cardiovascular disease. It is recommended that people take about 10,000 steps each day."* (Study: Lowering Physical Activity Impairs Glycemic Control in Healthy Volunteers, 2012).

● If a woman has developed Type 2 diabetes during pregnancy, or if they delivered a large baby.

If left untreated, it can lead to further health problems including blindness, amputation, heart attacks or other heart diseases, strokes and kidney disease.

What is Prediabetes?

Some of the alternative terms prediabetes has been known as in the past include, "early diabetes," "at risk for diabetes" and "borderline diabetes." As the terms indicate, prediabetes is a condition that comes prior to diabetes. When someone has prediabetes it means their blood glucose levels are very high but not high enough at this stage for it to be considered a diabetic condition. So while their body is still able to produce insulin and store sugar from the food and drink they consume for energy, it's not as effective as a healthy individual's body. The body tries to deal with this by increasing insulin production in a bid to get the blood glucose sugar up to the same level as it used to be. Eventually though, too much insulin is being used which leads to very little of it being produced. At this point, diabetes develops. The insulin in the body doesn't work as efficiently as it used to and therefore it causes the glucose levels to rise. If prediabetes remains undetected it can eventually lead to Type 2 diabetes as well as heart attacks and strokes.

What Causes Prediabetes?

As with Type 2 diabetes, prediabetes affects both children and adults and many factors have been known to cause it such as:

- **Genetics or a family history:** A person is known to be at a higher risk of developing prediabetes and Type 2 diabetes if a parent or sibling has it. However, could diet and lifestyle choices of the family as a whole be an underlying factor? Could this be why an individual is more prone to this condition rather than just "luck of the draw" when it comes to family genes?

- **A sedentary lifestyle:** If a person is inactive they are at a higher risk of developing prediabetes. Not only does exercise help to control weight, but it also allows for more glucose to be used as energy and the cells in the body to be more sensitive to insulin. We will delve deeper into the benefits of exercise further in the book.

● **Weight, including excess abdominal fat:** Being overweight or obese puts a person at high risk of developing prediabetes. When there is too much fatty tissue, especially within the muscle area and around the skin of the abdomen area, your cells become more resistant to insulin. A large abdomen area can be a sign that your cells are resistant to insulin. For example, men who have a waist that's larger than 40 inches are at a higher risk of being insulin resistant as are women with a waist that measures more than 35 inches.

● **Age:** Both children and adults can develop prediabetes, however adults who are in their 40s and older tend to be at a higher risk for the same reasons they are for developing Type 2 diabetes. For example, they have been exposed to sugary foods for longer periods of time and have already developed deep unhealthy habits that are now part of their day to day lifestyle. Also, many adults, especially over the age of 45, don't exercise as much; they gain weight and lose muscle mass which can be a contributing factor.

● **Dietary habits:** A diet that puts stress on the body such as consuming processed foods, sugary drinks and too much red meat on a regular basis can lead to prediabetes.

- **Race:** People of certain ethnic backgrounds are more prone to prediabetes although the reasons do not seem to be known by researchers. For instance, American scientists have found that African Americans, Asian Americans, Pacific Islanders, and Native Americans are at a higher risk.

- **Gestational diabetes:** This is another main type of diabetes and although it tends to go away once the mother has given birth, women who develop this condition during pregnancy are more likely to develop prediabetes as are their babies. Again, weight seems to play a role in the likelihood of developing it. For instance, a mother who gives birth to a baby that weighs over nine pounds at birth has an increased risk of developing prediabetes.

- **Sleep patterns:** Unsurprisingly, people who have irregular sleep patterns, including those who have sleep apnea, insomnia, work night shifts or often change shift working hours which may result in disruptive sleep, are also at a risk of developing prediabetes and Type 2 diabetes.

- **Polycystic Ovary Syndrome (PCOS):** This condition is a result of a hormonal imbalance which leads to excessive hair growth and weight gain (or obesity), and an irregular menstrual cycle. Insulin resistance is one of the key factors in this hormonal imbalance. Often times, women who have PCOS are prediabetic and can develop type 2 diabetes if dietary and lifestyle changes haven't yet been implemented.

● Other causes include, lower levels of 'good' cholesterol, high blood pressure, and higher levels of triglycerides.

In a nutshell, insulin resistance is the root cause for Type 2 diabetes. Why does the body become resistant to insulin? Some so-called experts claim it's still a 'mystery,' however the reason is very simple. According to Dr.Thomas Lordi (MD), an expert in both conventional and alternative medical practices, it comes down to what the pancreas has been exposed to: sugar and 'bad' fats. Too much of sugar and unhealthy fats cause the pancreas to become overtaxed.

Is Prediabetes Really Curable?

The straight answer is yes, prediabetes is curable. Since we already know that Type 2 diabetes can be reversed, it's also now understood that prediabetes can also be reversed and cured. However, many people, including healthcare professionals still believe that the only way this condition can be cured (or at best, managed) is by making a few lifestyle changes and taking prescription drugs. The question to ask is, *"Can prediabetes really be cured using natural methods?"*

Again, the answer is yes. It has been proven time and again in recent years that taking conventional medication is not necessary to cure prediabetes. It's actually important to take steps in reversing prediabetes through more natural methods because managing it solely with drugs can cause other problems over time.

The American Diabetes Association (ADA) often emphasizes that when people make a big lifestyle change, especially with their diet and exercise regime, after they have been diagnosed with prediabetes they can completely treat this condition and also prevent Type 2 diabetes from occurring:

"If you discover that you do have prediabetes, remember that it doesn't mean you'll develop type 2, particularly if you follow a treatment plan and a diet and exercise routine. Even small changes can have a huge impact on managing this disease or preventing it all together." (American Diabetes Association).

Chapter 2: Understanding Your Diagnosis

Often, when a person receives a diagnosis for a disease or any condition, they may feel afraid at first and then they are encouraged to 'fight' it. How many times have you watched a commercial for medicine that promises to 'fight' or "ward off" an illness? The truth is, it's not really about receiving a diagnosis and then feeling like you have to be at war with your body in order to 'fight' the condition or disease. This is one of the biggest misconceptions currently taking place in the healthcare industry.

There are many campaigns that urge people to act on 'fighting' *this* disease and "stand up to" *that* disease or the "war against" another. This idea of doing battle with the body can keep people feeling afraid and they hold the perception that they are powerless and at the mercy of their own bodies. It keeps people feeling separate from themselves, which is not the best state to be in if they are looking to balance any disease— *dis-ease*. When you start to truly understand your diagnosis and alter your perception, it becomes much easier to make changes. There is a saying, *"Prediabetes is a diagnosis. Taking control is a decision."*

Before we proceed to shift our perception on diagnosis, let's first look at the various symptoms you may receive.

27

What Will You Notice?

There can be symptoms for Type 2 diabetes, however when it comes to identifying the symptoms of *prediabetes*, many people don't have any symptoms at all. It's known as a "silent condition." The best way to find out if you have prediabetes is to have your blood sugar tested. This is especially important if you're prone to some of the lifestyle habits as mentioned in the previous chapter. For example, if you know you consume bad fats or sugary food and drinks frequently, and you feel you're living a sedentary lifestyle. Even if you believe that your lifestyle habits are balanced and healthy, it may be still worth having your blood sugar checked out.

Symptoms

If you can say 'yes' to the following then it's likely you have or could be at risk of having prediabetes:

- Are you over weight or considered to be obese?

- Do you live a sedentary lifestyle or do you feel you could be more physically active?

- Do you have high blood pressure?

- Do you have high cholesterol? This applies to having a higher amount of 'bad' fats and lower levels of 'good' fats.

- Have you given birth to a baby that weighs more than nine pounds?

- Do you have a close family member who has Type 2 diabetes?

There are some signs you may notice that indicate you could have gone from having prediabetes to Type 2 diabetes. These include:

- Constantly feeling thirstier than usual.

- Feeling more tired than you used to.

- Having to go to the restroom more often.

- Feeling hungrier than usual.

- Losing weight even though you're eating a lot.

- Blurred vision.

Insulin Resistance Symptoms

We have already discussed some of the factors associated with insulin resistance. However, here is a list so you can better understand if your body has developed a resistance to insulin.

- A large waist

- High blood pressure

- High blood sugar or high fasting blood sugar

- High triglycerides

- Low-density lipoprotein levels (HDLs)

- You may start developing dark patches on your skin (common areas are the knees, elbows, at the back of the neck and under the armpits).

How is Prediabetes Diagnosed?

If your GP suspects you may have prediabetes, they will likely want to perform tests. They may want to test your blood glucose sugar levels. There are three main tests that can be used to determine if you have prediabetes:

1. Hemoglobin A1c (HbA1c).

2. Oral Glucose Tolerance Test (OGTT).

3. Fasting Plasma Glucose Test (FPG).

Hemoglobin A1C Test (also known as HbA1c, and A1C)

There was a time when people relied on urine tests or pricking their finger to determine blood sugar levels. These two methods may have yielded accurate results—provided they were done in the moment, however they are not an effective way to measure someone's blood sugar overall. Blood glucose levels fluctuate throughout the day based on changes to your hormones, how active you've been, dietary intake, stress levels, etc. For instance, you may have high blood sugar levels in the early hours of the morning without realizing it.

The A1C test measures the amount of glucose that's bound to the hemoglobin (a protein that's located within red blood cells). Remember, we discussed earlier that if there is too much glucose being released into the blood then the pancreas will work harder to produce more insulin. This is what the A1C test measures—the amount of glucose in the blood, and if there is too much glucose that's binding to hemoglobin, you'll have a high A1C. If, however, the tests indicated that your hemoglobin are normal then your A1C will be normal too.

A1C tests measure a person's blood sugar levels over a two to three month period because that's how long the cells live. For instance, if your glucose levels were high two weeks ago and now they are normal, the A1C test will keep a record of the high levels as well as the level it is at now. It keeps a constant record over the three months. So, while it may not give an accurate reading of every moment in a given day, it does give a medical professional a good understanding of how your blood sugar level control has been over that time period.

However, it's worth keeping in mind that A1C tests can vary depending on a number of factors including:

- Changes to the temperature, equipment or sample handling

- Changes to hemoglobin or the red blood cells

- Changes to your blood glucose levels; they go up and down depending on a number factors as mentioned above, including sickness.

What Do the Percentages Indicate?

The National Institute of Diabetes and Digestive and Kidney Diseases have indicated that an A1C of 5.7 percent or below is 'normal.' If a person's reading shows 5.7 to 6.4 percent they have prediabetes and if it's 6.5 and above they have diabetes.

Please note that the A1C test isn't used to diagnose Type 1 diabetes, gestational diabetes or other conditions such as cystic fibrosis.

Fasting Plasma Glucose Test (FPG)

This is more likely to provide accurate results when it's done in the morning after having fasted for at least eight hours (no food or drink except for the occasion sips of water). A small sample of your blood is taken in order for the doctor to check your blood glucose levels. If your blood glucose levels are under 100 milligrams per deciliter (100mg/dL) then it's at a healthy level. If the tests indicate your blood glucose levels are between 100mg/dL and 125mg/dL then you have prediabetes, and anything over 126mg/dL means you have diabetes.

Oral Glucose Tolerance Test (OGTT)

As with FPG, when you take an Oral Glucose Tolerance Test (OGTT) you're required to fast for at least eight hours. On the day of the test, a medical professional will take some of your blood to test the glucose levels and then you will be given a glucose liquid to drink. After a couple of hours your blood glucose will be measured. If it measures anywhere between 140 to 199 mg/dL then you have prediabetes. If they measure 200mg/dL then you have diabetes. When you have the OGTT, it's likely you will hear healthcare professionals use the term "impaired glucose intolerance (IGT)," which is another way of saying 'prediabetes.'

You may wonder how accurate the tests are and whether each one can show different results. The National Institute of Diabetes and Digestive and Diseases (NIDDK) states that: *"In some people, a blood glucose test may show diabetes when an A1C test does not. The reverse can also occur—an A1C test may indicate diabetes even though a blood glucose test does not. Because of these differences in test results, health care professionals repeat tests before making a diagnosis.*

People with differing test results may be in an early stage of the disease, when blood glucose levels have not risen high enough to show up on every test. In this case, health care professionals may choose to follow the person closely and repeat the test in several months." (NIDDK).

Changing Your Perception on the Diagnosis

If your tests show high blood glucose levels and it's been confirmed that you have prediabetes or diabetes, there's no need to panic. The healthcare expert will likely provide you with recommendations on how to treat the condition which may include taking prescription drugs. Please be aware that conventional medicine is not the only answer.

Dr.Thomas Lodi, a conventional and alternative medical expert has stated that, *"Diagnosis is an opportunity to better educate yourself and learn to re-balance your body."* Earlier in the chapter, we acknowledged that when we have been diagnosed with a condition or dis-ease, it requires us to shift our perception of our bodies.

Rather than viewing your body as an enemy that's elusive and just does it's own thing whether you like it or not, it's important to understand that the body is always trying to find equilibrium, it *wants* to help you because it *is* you. We have devoted an entire chapter on the body's intelligence because it's so essential. However, for now we recommend that you start to adopt the perception that your diagnosis is an opportunity to re-learn how your body functions to serve you. It is your friend, not foe! Dr.Lodi has also stated that: *"People become insulin resistant which leads to Type II diabetes. You are not going to get rid of it because there is no 'it' to get rid of in this case.*

The way we have to look at this is the body becomes insulin resistant because it is getting overfed with sugar. **The body creates the resistance to protect itself".** (Lodi T).

We also recommend that you re-read the last sentence to help you make that shift in your perception. Dr.Lodi has taken, what some might consider to be a 'radical' view on Type 2 diabetes. He considers it to be an "eating disorder" due to the type of foods that are consumed frequently and over a period of time.

Now that we understand a diagnosis isn't as "doom and gloom" as it once was, it's time to explore ways insulin resistance can be reduced naturally.

Chapter 3: Three Effective Tips to Reduce Insulin Resistance Without Drugs

So far in this guide, we have come to the understanding that prediabetes and diabetes can be treated and reversed. We have also acknowledged that these conditions can be treated naturally and without conventional drugs. In the last chapter, we began to understand that the body works *for* us and *not against* us—this includes when we feel physical pain. Now that we know the body is on our side, despite how we have been conditioned to believe otherwise, it's time to set things into motion. Ideally, we want to do this by meeting our bodies at least half way. To do this is about more than just taking action with changing the diet and exercising. Yes, they are important and we'll discuss these components further in chapter four, however beforehand, we need to put ourselves in the right mental state. The following three tips run on from each other.

Tip 1: Why Your Mindset Matters

By developing the right mindset, it will make it easier to develop new habits and behaviors which will allow you to effectively implement the necessary strategies and methods that will bring about positive results. Although we're now at a time where more medical experts are beginning to understand that dramatic lifestyle changes are required to treat insulin resistance, there's often a key component that's missing. For instance, a doctor may tell you to change your diet and start becoming more physically active, but will they also tell you to change your mindset? Probably not! Before you go away to start changing your diet and planning your fitness regime, it's important to change your attitude so that it's in alignment with the new lifestyle you want. If you don't do this, you will likely find that after a few weeks (or even days), you revert back to the old habits that brought about the insulin resistance in the first place. Even if you don't revert back straight away, you may find it a chore (and a bore) to adopt the new lifestyle changes. It could lead to resentment over time, which will end up being stressful—not what we want!

Your mind is connected to your body and since the two are not separate, it's important that they work together in harmony rather than against each other. For example, your body may want to consume certain types of foods or engage in a particular activity that will help to restore the insulin balance. Your mind, however, due to years of eating certain foods that you may be addicted to, may want something else. Perhaps you're not open to the idea of carrying out an activity because you may perceive it to be too 'challenging.' If so, your mind will 'win' and you won't take the necessary steps to make the healthier choices. This is mind over matter.

So how can you adopt a mindset that will assist in reducing insulin resistance?

1. **Be accountable:** This isn't about beating yourself up over choices you've made—doing that will only place further stress on your body. Instead, it's a good idea to hold yourself accountable for past choices and present ones. When you acknowledge that responsibility for your health is ultimately down to you, it allows you to take back your power (which you probably gave away to others due to social conditioning).

2. **Education:** Ideally, it's advised that you be open to learning as much as you can about how your pancreas works and the impact your lifestyle choices have on the body. You're already reading this guide which means you care deeply about becoming more informed. There is a "further resources" section at the back of the book which will help you to increase your knowledge. By educating

yourself you're actually retraining your mind to focus on reducing insulin resistance.

3. **Set goals and make a plan:** It would be a good idea to think about your goals and then write them down. There are a number of ways you can go about this. For example, you could make SMART goals (S*pecific, Measurable, Attainable/Achievable, Realistic/Relevant,* and *Time-based/Timely*). Alternatively, you could simply write down your short-term and long-term goals and what action steps you intend to take. Having clear goals in mind and writing them down are key. You also want to make a plan, which is based on your goals. By the time you read this guide you will have clear goals and a plan to work with. Your plan might include a meal plan and chapter eight will help you with that.

Writing down your goals allows your mind to work on ways to help you achieve them. A study carried out by Professor Gail Matthews, PHD at the Dominican University of California has found that writing down goals increases your chances of reaching them. Remember, your body is trying it's best to maintain balance and harmony within the system and by writing down your goals, such as your desire to reduce insulin resistance, you're already allowing your mind to be on the same 'page' as your body.

4. **Be committed:** If you're not committed to rebuilding a healthy body then it won't happen. There may be times when you just don't feel like exercising or reaching out for a healthier snack, and although we don't condone you go against your body's wishes, if you don't remain committed and have some amount of discipline, it will be very difficult for you to reduce insulin resistance. Again, if you write down what you're committed to this will help to reinforce it in your mind.

Tip 2: Improving Your Habits and Behaviors for Success

As your mindset starts to alter, you will find that carrying out new habits and behaviors will come more naturally to you. It may not happen straight away but eventually it will. The way to improve your habits and behaviors include:

1. Creating a plan of action (daily, weekly and monthly or quarterly) and making sure you *act* on it everyday.

2. We have mentioned that in order to reverse diabetes or prediabetes big lifestyle changes are required. However, if you aren't 100% sure you can implement those changes immediately, you can always take smaller steps and then build on them. For instance, if it's your goal to exercise for 45 minutes every day but you have previously been inactive, then it's best to start with five minutes a day and then build from there.

3. Have an accountability friend. Sometimes it can be difficult to motivate ourselves, especially when old thought patterns and behaviors try to creep back in. It can be powerful to have someone in our lives who will help to hold us accountable. Studies have shown that having social support or having

someone who can help us to keep track of our goals is very beneficial and yields powerful results. Perhaps you could find someone else who also has a goal to reduce their insulin resistance and be each other's accountability buddy. You can agree to meet up or speak every week or month to make sure you're both staying on top of goals. Here are some ways you can go about reaching out for support:

❖ Exercise with a family member, friend, colleague or acquaintance.

❖ Find a support group. If you can't find any suitable groups in your area you can always start a group or check online. There are groups such as DietBet. You may want to start or find a group that deals specifically with reducing insulin resistance using natural methods.

❖ Your accountability buddy doesn't have to be someone who has similar goals to you (although we think it would really benefit).

4. Taking action is the key. Having goals and a plan of action is important. Changing your mindset is crucial. However, you must take action consistently. Again, please remember

that you don't have to take massive action straight away, especially if you strongly suspect you will quit after a few days. You can always take baby steps with your behavioral changes and as they become new habits you will find they come naturally to you. Then, you can start to introduce more changes. Again, *consistency* is key. It has been a *consistent* effort on your part with lifestyle habits that have likely created the insulin resistance in the first place (no blame) so there's no reason why you cannot start again with alternative choices.

Tip 3: Ways to Adopt and Maintain a Healthier Lifestyle

We will be discussing in detail exactly how to change your lifestyle to reverse prediabetes or diabetes in the upcoming chapters. In this section, we want to provide you with an overview of the ways you can adopt a healthier lifestyle to reduce insulin resistance naturally:

1. **Intermittent fasting.** It has been used throughout history and animals who live in the wild do it naturally. They don't eat three meals a day plus a lot of sugary snacks in between. Instead, they may eat for two or three days and then go up to a week without eating. When we are not eating, our bodies have the opportunity to cleanse itself. Unfortunately, with our unconscious habits, it doesn't really get that chance. Intermittent fasting involves a period of fasting and non-fasting and is known to decrease insulin levels. According to Dr.Jason Fung (MD) who is one of the world's leading experts on intermittent fasting for treating Type 2 diabetes, intermittent fasting drops the insulin levels and helps the body to change the demand for it: *"If you become very insulin resistant, then your insulin levels are up all the time, your body is always trying to shove the energy into the fat cells, and then you feel cold and tired and lousy. That's the*

real problem. Resistance really depends on two things. It's not simply the high levels, but it's the persistence of those levels. What people have realized is that the insulin resistance, because it depends on those two things, a period of time where you can get your insulin levels very low is going to break that resistance because it breaks that persistence. Not simply the levels, but the persistence of those levels." (Fung J).

2. **Become more active**—even if it's just walking more. If you don't feel like breaking out a sweat, rather than do nothing at all you could instead go for a brisk walk—even for just half an hour. If you're short on time, why not jump rope for 10 to 15 minutes? By finding ways to increase your activity even if you're busy or not feeling up to it, you can keep the momentum going. If you don't exercise on a regular basis, your body is unable to properly remove the waste that can build up around your cells.

3. **Do something you enjoy** on a daily or weekly basis to help keep your spirits up so you feel motivated with the new lifestyle change. Sometimes, when we break old habits, it can be a bit uncomfortable at first and may lead some people to feel discouraged or agitated, but if you schedule in some "fun time" to do an activity that brings you joy, it

can make all the difference. Ideally, if your fun time can include doing something creative or active such as playing with your kids in the park, all the better!

Chapter 4: How to Defend Yourself from Type 2 Diabetes

So far, this guide has mentioned that diet, exercise and stress management are important factors in reversing Type 2 diabetes. Now we are going to explore each one in detail so you have a good understanding of how you can introduce these changes into your life. The suggestions in this chapter applies to both children and adults.

Why Your Diet is Important

We mentioned earlier that the body is intelligent and is always doing it's best to find balance even if it means causing what you may perceive to be pain and suffering. If you have been eating too much of the wrong foods then it will try it's best to work with what you give it. Once you start to alter your diet so that your body is being nourished with what it truly requires, it can more easily get back into balance. By adopting a diet that will prevent Type 2 diabetes, your pancreas will feel relieved!

Foods to Avoid

You want to avoid foods that are high on the glycemic index such as white bread and pasta because they increase blood pressure. Limit alcohol intake and ideally stop smoking. We have mentioned in this guide that sugary foods cause insulin resistance and the blood to store too much glucose. In chapters six and seven we will delve deeper into foods to avoid and what to eat. Don't feel too disappointed though as you will discover in upcoming chapters that there are plenty of delicious healthy alternatives to choose from. Many people find that once they have cut out unhealthy foods and their bodies have detoxed from sugar completely, their taste buds alter to such an extent that addictions complete vanish!

Foods to Eat

You want to eat foods that are found in certain food groups so your body receives everything it needs to repair. Diets that are known to help include raw vegan plant-based diet that is low in carbohydrates and the ketogenic diet. Both of which we will discuss further. For now, here is a list of foods you want to incorporate into your diet:

Vegetables (organic and fresh is ideal)

Vegetables have less impact on blood glucose levels than most fruits (which *may* need to be avoided).

Fruits (organic and fresh is ideal)

As mentioned above, certain fruits should be avoided

as they will increase blood glucose levels. Although there are researchers who believe that some of these fruits are actually good at preventing diabetes. Perhaps you want to avoid them in the beginning and then later, you can slowly re-introduce them into your diet. Go with what feels right for you.

Nuts, grains and seeds (provided you are not allergic)

Overall, they help to manage your insulin levels as they are anti-inflammatory and low on the glycemic index.

Oily Fish

Oily fish contains high amounts of Omega 3, which helps to protect the heart from heart disease. If you can, try and eat fresh fish once or twice a week, or at the very least take Omega 3 fish oil as a supplement.

Your Exercise Regime

There is no one-size-fits-all when it comes to choosing an exercise regime. You will need to find one that's right for you. Some experts have suggested that losing one to two pounds a week is ideal. However, please bare in mind that everyone's metabolism works differently and while some people may lose two pounds a week, it may take longer for others to lose weight.

Choosing an Exercise Regime That's Right For You

Dr.Thomas Lodi has suggested that simple gentle movement such as walking, riding a bike or light jogging can do wonders. It's not necessary to do a 45 minute vigorous exercise routine everyday, unless you feel drawn to do that. If you have mainly lived a sedentary lifestyle for many years, then suddenly starting off your new exercise regime with 45, 60, or 90 minutes of high intensity may not be helpful. You're more likely to lose momentum, burn yourself out or just resent having to do it. Instead, find things that you'll enjoy and commit to doing those weekly. You can always alternate your exercise regime. For instance, one week you could focus on one or two types of exercises and then switch it up the following week. Eventually, you may want to have a mixture of the following three:

Aerobic exercise

This involves cardio to get the heart pumping fast and the blood flowing. Unless you have a lot of experience in being very physically active, it's a good idea to not go overboard with aerobic as you could increase the risk of muscle fatigue. Instead, aim for two or three times a week at 30 minutes each or even 10 minutes in the morning and 10 at night. Make it fun! Examples of aerobic exercises are:

- Cycling

- Swimming

- Jogging/running

- Skipping

- Dancing

- Walking (briskly)

- Badminton/Tennis

- Stationary cycling (using a machine)

Strength exercise/resistance training

Strength training and resistance training involves using weights like dumbbells or a kettlebell (to name a few) to build muscle strength. It doesn't always have to involve weights as there are certain exercise routines that don't require any equipment. Since strength exercises help to build muscle instead of fat, it's great at helping people who are at risk of having, or have already developed Type 2 diabetes. It helps to control their glucose because the muscles require plenty of it.

If you choose to lift weights then approximately 20 minutes two or three times a week is fine. However, you must always listen to your body.

Examples of strength/resistance training includes:

● Planks

● Sit-ups

● Press-ups

● Kettlebell

● Bench press

● Single arm dumbbell

● Squats

● Leg press

High Intensity Interval Training (HIIT)

This type of exercise includes short periods of cardiovascular activity (between 20 seconds to a minute or two) followed by rest periods in between. This differs from a long jog, which is a form of steady-state exercise (SSE) where you reserve your energy levels so that you can complete the run. With HIIT, during short bursts of cardiovascular activity, you must give it all you've got to really get the heart pumping fast, and then you *must* rest to get the heart rate back down.

Studies have shown that HIIT is very effective at eliminating fat and regulating insulin levels. A study carried out on forty-five women, which was published in the International Journal of Obesity, has concluded that: *"HIIE (High Intensity Interval Exercise) three times per week for 15 weeks compared to the same frequency of SSE exercise was associated with significant reductions in total body fat, subcutaneous leg and trunk fat, and insulin resistance in young women."* (Trapp EG, 2008).

HIIT workouts can often involve the use of your body's weight. For example, push-ups, sit-ups, burpees, weightlifting, etc. Remember, the recovery period in between each interval is just as important because it helps to prepare the body for the next burst of cardio activity. The intention is that you work really hard, take a rest and then work really hard again. HITT is known to be generally suitable for everyone and it does provide a number of other benefits including:

- Improves your mental and emotional well-being.

- Can be done in as little as 10 minute, which is great if you're having a busy day.

- It's a very flexible routine and there are many exercises you can choose from.

- It's ideal for people who have low energy levels (many people with insulin resistance or diabetes do).

- It can continue to burn calories for hours after you have finished exercising.

- It can be just as (if not more) effective as doing long-form exercise.

HIIT is not to everyone's taste and it's important you access your body's needs first.

Flexibility exercise

This includes low-intensity exercise and encourages your muscles and joints to work properly which then makes your exercise session much easier. For instance, you want to make sure you warm up before exercise and cool down afterwards. Often, when we start to exercise (especially when we haven't done it for a while) our joints and muscles can feel very sore for even a few days after. If you plan to exercise daily or a few times a week then trying to do that when you already have existing joint or muscle pain can put you at a greater risk of developing muscle fatigue or other injuries. Flexibility exercises can yield powerful results and can get the heart pumping due to the effort required to control joints and muscles.

Here are some different forms of flexibility exercise you may choose to take up:

- Tai Chi

- Pilates

- Yoga

- Lifting weights

- Hiking

- Dancing

- Walking up steps

The best thing to do is create a plan or contact your local gym if you're after a trainer, and see what feels right for you. You may have to experiment with some exercises if you aren't sure what you'd like to do. The important thing is to get started with moving your body.

Stress Management

Ways to Reduce Stress

You will find that changing your diet and becoming more physically active will help to reduce stress. As you begin to reduce or eliminate refined foods from your diet you will start to feel happier, have more energy and a positive outlook on life. There are numerous studies that show a high sugar intake increases the risk of depression. This is hardly surprising considering how stressful the body becomes when we eat the wrong types of food and don't allow ourselves to be active. This affects our hormones, and in particular serotonin, which is responsible for our mood and aggression. Serotonin isn't just a neurotransmitter that's located in the brain, it's also found in our central nervous system and the pancreas.

In addition to changing your diet and becoming more physically active, it's essential that you prioritize managing your stress levels, even if it means taking just five minutes a day to do something that will help keep you calm and centered.

Mindfulness

Mindfulness is a practice that involves being aware of what's taking place in the present moment without being in judgement. It has been proven by scientists to be effective at reducing stress and encouraging a sense of well-being. Many employers now hire mindfulness coaches to teach employees on how to practice this skill, which has been used by Buddhists throughout history. Since mindfulness is known to help with improving health, mindset, behavior, and habits, it's worth considering it as part of your daily care. Other known specific benefits include:

- Heightening your intuition (essential if you're to start listening to your body's messages).
- Deepening your appreciation for life.
- Improving sleep.
- Helping to lower your blood pressure.
- Helping to treat heart disease.
- Helping to treat eating disorders.
- Helping to treat obsessive-compulsive disorder (OCD).
- Alleviating depression and anxiety.
- Helping to reduce chronic pain.

There are a number of mindfulness techniques you can use such as meditation. You can start by sitting somewhere quietly and observing your breathing. If you like, chant a mantra or a word to help bring your awareness into the present moment.

Journaling

We mentioned in the last chapter how writing down your goals is a powerful way to help bring about results. Writing in general is beneficial, especially when you're writing down your thoughts. We would encourage you to get into the habit of jotting down your thoughts, insights, ideas, frustrations, etc. You may find that as your body starts to cleanse itself from sugary foods and your mood improves, your thoughts will become clearer. Perhaps you may receive profound dreams—it might be worth having a dream journal too, if that's the case.

Journaling is a great way to release stress and any pent up emotion as you are acknowledging situations and expressing yourself, even if it's just on paper and you never vocalize it to anyone else. If you really don't like the idea of writing, you could always record your thoughts using a dictaphone.

Creativity

Creativity comes in many different forms so have a think about what you would like to do. Perhaps you like the idea of playing a musical instrument or listening to music. Maybe you used to enjoy dancing and want to get back into that (great way to exercise too). Do you love the idea of spending time with your grandchildren and creating a scrapbook or building something? Perhaps you like to draw, paint, build Lego with your children, write stories, color in pictures or get involved in crafts and hobbies. The ideas are limitless, which means you don't have to do a specific activity either. Even just getting some play dough and making shapes can help to alleviate stress.

Being in Nature

This is part of being mindful as it gives you the opportunity to really observe your surroundings and just be present. Being in nature allows you to get some exercise and plenty of oxygen. You don't have to go far—a stroll to your nearest park or wood will do wonders. Studies have shown that just 20 minutes of being in nature can cause cortisol levels to drop.

Spending Time With Loved Ones

Here are some reasons why it's good to spend time with friends and family:

- Boosts your confidence and self-esteem.
- Reduces stress.
- Helps you to make more positive choices.
- More likely to live longer.

In addition to the above, it's also important that you get your blood tested regularly so you are better able to monitor it and see if there are any further changes you need to make to your diet, exercise regime or stress management.

Chapter 5: A New Approach to Diabetes

If you've already started to do your own research on diabetes prior to reading this guide, you may have noticed that there appears to be conflicting information on what causes diabetes and how to treat it. As we have already mentioned, there are still a number of medical health professionals who believe that diabetes cannot be reversed, only controlled to a certain degree. There are medical scientists who still believe it's a complete mystery as to how insulin resistance and Type 2 diabetes can occur. However, *we* are now aware that:

a) Type 2 diabetes can indeed be prevented as well as reversed; and

b) It's no longer a mystery as to why people develop insulin resistance and diabetes.

According to Dr.Sarah Hallberg, a Medical Director at IU Health Arnett, everything we consume contains either fats, carbohydrates or proteins. Each one impacts our glucose and insulin levels differently. During a Tedx Talk Dr.Hallbert presented a graph that shows carbohydrates have the highest impact on our insulin and blood glucose levels which makes them rise in a short period of time.

The graph also shows that when we eat protein, it doesn't have such a dramatic impact, but what's interesting is that when we consume fats, they have very little to no impact. These results play a significant role in how we choose to move forward with a new approach to diabetes. Before we discuss new approaches that cutting edge medical experts are advocating, let's first acknowledge how Type 2 diabetes has been dealt with in the past.

How Type 2 Diabetes Has Been Treated in the Past

Many people consume food in the following manner:

1. They eat a large meal full of carbohydrates, and eat so much too quickly that the body doesn't have a chance to register that it's full.

2. The person feels 'overstuffed' and bloated.

3. An hour or two later they feel hungry again and wonder what else they could eat. Why are they hungry again? Because the carbohydrates they ate have caused insulin and blood glucose levels to spike quickly. Dr.Hallberg says that this *"triggers hunger, fat storage, and cravings."* (Hallberg 2015). This is an ongoing cycle, especially if a person is insulin resistant in the first place. It means they're always

hungry and despite eating, their bodies are actually starving!

4. The advice people were receiving in the past was very damaging and counter-intuitive. For instance, Dr. Hallberg discussed how patients with Type 2 diabetes have been told to consume 40 to 65 grams of carbohydrates with *every* meal, plus snacks! She has suggested that Type 2 diabetes is caused by consuming too many carbohydrates and insulin resistance is triggered due to an intolerance of carbohydrates. So, the cycle that's going on in relation to the advice people receive consists of eating carbohydrates, and therefore you must take diabetic medication. Then eat more carbohydrates (due to the side effects of the medication), and the cycle continues. These are the guidelines given from healthcare associates, Unfortunately, in the guidelines it doesn't stipulate how to reverse Type 2 diabetes.

What may be surprising to many people is that it's possible we don't actually need carbohydrates. Dr. Hallerberg has discussed that we don't need them at all. Instead what the body requires are essential amino acids (protein) and essential fatty acids. So the approach that the medical profession has been taking—the outdated approach—is for patients with Type 2 diabetes to consume over half of their daily energy intake through carbohydrates.

On the other hand, Dr. Neal Barnard, a Clinical Researcher and founder of the Physicians Committee for Responsible Medicine (PCRM) has stated that there was a time when medical professionals were advising patients to not eat anything that turns into sugars such as bread, pasta, rice, fruit, potatoes, and other carbohydrates, and also they were to lower their calories. In addition, they had to use needles and inject insulin. We can see the conflicting advice people have been given throughout the years. It is any wonder that the amount of people who have pre-diabetes or diabetes has risen so dramatically?

Dr. Barnard argues that there have been two scientific discoveries. The first is that cultures throughout the world who are known to have very low rates of diabetes don't have the type of diet that people with Type 2 diabetes in the USA are prescribed. For instance, in Japan they actually eat white rice and noodles frequently. The second discovery is that when scientists have looked inside of muscle cells where glucose should be found, for people with Type 2 diabetes they find fat. This is what makes it difficult or impossible for glucose to enter the cells, according to Dr. Barnard. In 2003, he carried out research on 99 people, having them eat as much as they wanted but cut out fat from the diet. This meant they couldn't consume animal products and they could only eat low amounts of vegetable oils. His research concluded that Type 2 diabetes can be reversed by eliminating fats, mainly animal fats. Dr. Barnard's argument is that the human body has not evolved to handle animal fats and meats and by removing them from our diet and consuming plant-based foods, we can reverse Type 2 diabetes and other diseases.

So, what are the new approaches to treating this disease?

New Approaches to Treating Diabetes

There we have it: Two medical experts with completely different views on how to treat diabetes. This isn't uncommon, but what's interesting is that both have evidence to back up their claims which then raises the question, is there only one 'right' way to reverse diabetes or are there multiple ways depending on the needs of a person's body?

While Dr.Hallberg and Dr.Barnard have new approaches on Type 2 diabetes, both seem to contradict the other. However, since this guide is about helping you to become more informed so that you are in a place to make choices based on your body's needs, we will discuss both approaches as they each make valid points. When it comes to diet and exercise, there isn't a one-size-fits-all, so it's important to be open to different perceptions so we can find one that works well for us.

Approach 1: Eat Your Fats! (Dr.Sarah Hallberg)

Dr.Hallberg's approach to treating diabetes is to ensure that healthcare organizations/associations make it clear in their guidelines that Type 2 diabetes can be reversed. She believes that people should be given practical steps to do it. This is what Hallberg recommends:

1. Cutting out carbohydrates from the diet or eat with them being the minority of the diet. Her argument is that when her patients cut down on carbohydrates, their blood glucose levels go down so they don't need as much insulin which then begins to decrease quickly.

Here are her findings:

"A young [woman] who had an almost twenty year history of Type 2 diabetes...her diabetes was way out of control, this despite the fact that she was on multiple medications including, almost 300 units of insulin that was being injected into her continuously every day via a pump. We put her on a low carb diet and now let's fast forward four months. She lost weight—yes—but better than that, sick no more. Her blood sugar levels were now normal all of the time, this on...no diabetes medication. Gone was the 300 units of insulin, no more insulin pump. No more pricking her finger multiple times each day. No more

diabetes. One of the greatest joys of my job is to be able to tell a patient like this that they no longer have diabetes...So, are they cured? Is this a miracle?...Cured would imply that it can't come back and if they start eating excessive carbs again it will, so no not cured. But, they don't have diabetes any longer. It's resolved and it can stay that way as long as we keep away the cause." (Hallberg 2015).

A low carbohydrate diet doesn't mean zero carbohydrates, nor does it mean consuming high amounts of protein. Hallberg's patients eat plenty of fat as it's the *only* macronutrient out of the three (carbohydrates and protein being the other two) that will keep the insulin and blood glucose levels down. So, the requirements of this approach include:

- Avoiding foods that are labelled as 'fat-free,' 'low fat' or 'light.' Dr.Hallberg has emphasized that if fat has been taken out of the food then it's been replaced with carbohydrates and/or chemicals.
- Eat real, whole foods rather than refined foods.
- Don't eat any foods you don't like.
- Eat when you are hungry and when you're not hungry, don't eat, despite what the time is.
- Avoid grains, potatoes, and sugar.

So, this new approach is about the healthcare professional and the patient having the goal to reverse the disease and reduce or be able to eliminate medication. This brings up the question as to why more medical professionals are not suggesting a low carbohydrate, high fat diet. Unfortunately, the reason is quite cynical. There are a couple of reasons that Dr.Hallberg has identified:

1. The **status quo** is hard to break as there are a number of agendas taking place within the medical professional field. Many healthcare experts feel frustrated that the advice of "cut out fats" is still being perpetuated as they believe this concept is outdated.

2. "There is a lot of **money** to be made by keeping you sick," according to Dr.Hallberg.

The solution in Dr.Hallberg's clinic is to stop using medicine to treat the disease and instead take a sensible approach with our food, going off the latest findings.

Approach 2: Cut Out Fats! (Dr. Neal Barnard)

Dr. Barnard's view is that fats, especially animal fats should be cut out of the diet and we are better off sticking to the diet that our bodies have evolved for: plant-based foods. He argues that Americans eat too many animals (approximately one million per hour).

His vision includes people reducing their animal meat intake and having farmers just sell beans, fruit and vegetables instead of meat. When Dr.Barnard carried out a study in 2003, he discovered that when participants ate a plant-based diet, their blood sugar levels were controlled as much as three times more effectively than when they were eating a diet that has previously been recommended to people with Type 2 diabetes. His argument is that when people eat a diet that is high in fatty foods, it causes fat to build up in the cells, which prevents insulin from being able to distribute glucose from our blood into the cells.

Dr.Barnard's new approach to tackling diabetes is as follows:

1. Eat a plant-based diet that's full of fruits, vegetables, whole grains, and legumes.

2. Limit high food fats such as oils and animal fats.

3. Consume foods that are low on the GI Index such as oats, sweet potatoes, and beans.

4. Consume about 40 grams of fiber a day. Dr.Barnard's findings suggest that eating fiber helps to control blood glucose levels.

Both medical experts do seem to have one thing in common: A belief that Type 2 diabetes can be reversed and without the need for medication. One new approach is to consume high fats and another new approach is to reduce them. Is this proof that there is more than one way to treat diabetes naturally? It could depend on a person's blood type, health history, lifestyle, and other factors playing a role in determining what diet will be most effective for them. Perhaps the biggest takeaway from this chapter is that there are (natural) options available and if you aren't drawn to a particular method, you can always try another.

A Short message from the Author:

Hey, are you enjoying the book? I'd love to hear your thoughts!

Many readers do not know how hard reviews are to come by, and how much they help an author.

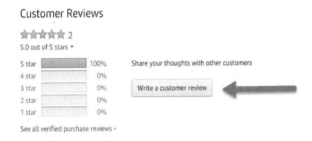

I would be incredibly thankful if you could take just 60 seconds to write a brief review on Amazon, even if it's just a few sentences!

Your review will genuinely make a difference for me and help gain exposure for my work.

Thank you for taking the time to share your thoughts!

Chapter 6: Reverse Diabetes in Eight Weeks

We must emphasize that while diabetes can be reversed within a matter of weeks, a suitable diet must be followed. For instance, if you decide to adopt a diet that consists of low fats then it's no good consuming low fat meals that are highly processed. If you are going to follow a plant-based diet that is low in fat then it's no use in following it once or twice a week and then the rest of the time eating cooked high fatty, processed foods. This approach will cause more damage. Whether you're pre-diabetic or have already been diagnosed with Type 2 diabetes, it's important you have a plan and follow it. This is why having the right mindset is important.

We're going to take into account the extensive research undertaken by cutting-edge medical professionals and focus on the two new approaches mentioned in the previous chapter, to reverse diabetes. In this chapter we will explore a plant-based diet with a ration of 80/20: 80 percent being raw vegan food and 20 percent being cooked. Then, in chapter seven we will focus on a low carbohydrate, high fat diet, which is known as the ketogenic diet. Unlike the old approaches to dealing with Type 2 diabetes, these two new ones can provide results within eight weeks.

How Diabetes Can be Reversed in Eight Weeks

Plant-Based Diets

Dr.Barnard's Plant-Based Diet Approach

An article published on Dr.Neal Barnard's website states that:

"The old approach recommended cutting down on carbohydrates. It's true that overly processed carbohydrates—those made with sugar or white flour, for example—are poor choices. However, delicious unprocessed or minimally processed foods, such as potatoes, rice, oats, beans, pasta, fruit, and vegetables, were the main part of the diet in countries where people were traditionally fit and trim and where diabetes was rare. Unfortunately, highly processed carbohydrates and affordable meat and cheese dishes have moved in, and now we have a worldwide type 2 diabetes epidemic.

Diet and Diabetes:

Recipes for Success

A low-fat vegetarian approach recognizes that whole-food carbohydrates are fine; it's the fat in our diets that is the problem. New information suggests that fat in animal products and oils interferes with insulin's ability to move glucose into the cells. Eating less fat reduces body fat. Less body fat allows insulin to do its job. However, choosing skinless chicken, skim milk, and baked fish is not enough of a change for most people to beat diabetes." (Physicians Committee For Responsible Medicine).

Dr.Barnard's approach includes a diet that's built around the following foods (your "Power Plate"):

1. Fruits

2. Grains

3. Legumes (including beans, lentils and peas)

4. Vegetables

He advises that you drink plenty of water and you can also snack on a handful of nuts and seeds once a day. As this is a vegan diet, Barnard stresses it's important to remember that animal products must be avoided since they contain the type of fat (saturated fat) that can cause heart disease and other health problems. Animal products to avoid include the following:

● Red meats (beef, lamb and pork).

● Poultry (chicken, turkey, duck and geese, etc).

- Dairy products (eggs, milk, cheese, butter, yoghurt).

- Vegetable oils and other foods that contain high fats (foods that have been fried in oil, not too many nuts including peanut butter, limit avocados and olives).

- Sugary foods such as puffed cereals and corn flakes, white and wheat breads.

Opt for foods with a low GI. These include:

- Breads such as whole wheat, rye, sourdough, multigrain, pumpernickel, pitta, and tortillas.

- White wheat pasta.

- Oats.

- Cereals such as muesli, oatmeal (rolled or steel-cut), and bran.

- Grains such as quinoa, couscous, and rice.

Surprisingly, foods such as white wheat pasta are lower in GI, along with sweet potatoes, corn, butter beans, and yams.

Include fiber into the diet (approximately 40 grams a day). Foods that contain high fiber include vegetables, whole grains and beans. Remember to start small as your bowel movements are likely to change.

An example of a meal plan for a day could include:

Breakfast: Fresh Fruit or All Bran with non-fat rice milk.

Lunch: A salad full of mixed vegetables with fat-free dressing or lemon juice.

Dinner: A vegetable stir-fry with a low-fat stir fry sauce, served with pasta or rice.

Snack: Soup or tortilla chips with salsa dip.

Dr.Lodi's Plant-Based Diet Approach

Dr.Lodi argues that Type 2 diabetes is the body's way of trying to balance and heal itself. He states:

"...Your body is doing this to protect you. Keep in mind there is no such thing as diseases. 'Diseases' are the body trying to maintain the integrity of the organism. What we need to do is get rid of the reason why the body is doing that...The body is resistant because there is too much of this glucose. So, stop eating the glucose. As a matter of fact, if you are a

Type 2 diabetic, all you have to do is for 21 days just eat raw vegan food...which is nuts, seeds, vegetables and don't eat the fruit. If you are going to eat the fruit eat some berries, some apples—for now, for the first 21 days, but mostly vegetables...by the end of the 21 days you will be off all medication...and this happens 100% of the time. Once you are off that medication, then you can start to play around and modify your diet..." (Lodi 2015).

Dr.Lodi advises that it's important to train your body to get full on foods that are packed with nutrients so that you won't crave the wrong type of foods. When we eat foods that are full of starches and are processed, they never satisfy the body. He emphasizes that this is why many people are always looking for a snack, even after consuming a large meal. The craving for snacks is your body's way of saying, "I'm not satisfied. I haven't received what I truly need to function at my best."

Lodi's perception of Type 2 diabetes is that it's nothing more than an eating disorder than can be rectified. He suggests that if you want to stay on track with this type of diet, it's important to 'fool' yourself into not feeling hungry. If you feel hungry or tired, it's much easier to be swayed off the diet as you're more likely to reach for sugary snacks and other processed foods to get that 'hit.' The way to help you stay on track, Lodi advises getting a handful of nuts and seeds, soak them overnight and then in the morning use a paper towel to remove access moisture and then put them in a tupperware and carry it with you everywhere you go. By snacking on these slightly sprouted nuts and seeds it will prevent you from feeling hungry and diminish the cravings for the wrong types of food.

Lodi also advises not eating a meal three hours before you go to bed as your sleep will not be as restful due to your body going through the digestive process. If you go to bed feeling very full, there is a higher risk of you waking up with gastric irritation which may seem like hunger. In his diabetes program at The LifeCo, the four ways to recover from Type 2 diabetes are through diet, detoxing the body, natural therapies and a healing environment.

Detoxing the body

Since your body is likely to be full of toxins, due to years of processed foods, cleansing out the system with a liquid detox diet for a couple of weeks can help to regulate blood sugar levels, eliminate toxins and balance out your hormones. The fast can consist of water fasting or green juice.

Lodi recommends a water fast as the best liquid detox because *"it's the only cure handed down by nature. When an animal is sick they stop eating and just drink water—they don't drink a lot, but just enough to keep them hydrated."* (Lodi 2015).

During the first three days of a water fast, the body should use up the stored glucose and then after that the glucose levels should go down and your ketones (substances that are produced in the liver) will go up. When you continue on the water fasting diet, the ketone/glucose ratio should start to balance itself out to less than 1.0. Dr.Lodi advises that this happens on a water fast. This ratio is also what we aim for on the ketogenic diet (chapter seven). He believes that water fasting is the "ultimate ketogenic diet." This fasting gives the body an opportunity to rest from the digestive process and start to cleanse and renew itself.

Diet

Once your blood sugar levels have reduced due to detoxing, a diet that involves consuming mostly raw vegan food, with a low carbohydrate intake is the next step. Lodi advises having long gaps in between your first meal and the last—18 hours—is important because during the long gap, your sugar reducing hormone levels will decrease.

Natural therapies

To aid the body in cleansing, therapies such as enemas and colon hydrotherapy helps to release toxins through the colon. Massages, infrared sauna or steam baths help to release toxins through the skin (the body's largest organ).

Exercise

Dr.Lodi believes that exercise is important but it doesn't need to be strenuous. The goal is to increase your cardio fitness and that could just be walking more than you usually do or some light jogging.

The right environment

This can include joining a support group or finding an accountability partner (as mentioned in chapter four). The right environment can also mean sometimes finding somewhere that's peaceful so you can unwind, if only for 30 minutes.

Other methods to apply during these critical weeks

- Prayer and/or meditation.
- Plenty of sleep.
- Guided visualization.

Other healthcare professionals who have had success with helping their patients to reverse Type 2 diabetes within weeks include Dr.Sandita Shah and Dr.Gabriel Cousens. Both of which have written books on reversing Type 2 diabetes within 30 days by adopting a plant-based diet.

Chapter 7: The Benefits of the Ketogenic Diet

Now it's time to discuss the other new approach to treating Type 2 diabetes: Low carbohydrates and high fat. The ketogenic diet is a great example of this.

The liver produces two substances from fat and they are classed as ketones. They can either be made from fat that is already stored in the body or from fat that we eat (which is through the blood after we've digested the food). These fats are quite difficult to transport as they are contained in lipoprotein particles. These lipoprotein particles are what is measured when we are monitoring cholesterol levels (triglycerides, etc). It has been discovered through research that when the fat in the liver is turned into ketones, you don't need to worry about lipoproteins because ketones are able to float through the blood and into cells easily. Therefore, they are a more efficient fuel for the body to use. The wonderful thing is that there are plenty of ketones in the blood, they can feed the brain, your muscles and heart, as well as other things.

What's even more exciting is that ketones talk to our genes, especially the ones that are responsible for "free radicals" or "oxidative stress," known to be the root cause of Type 2 diabetes, heart disease, irritable bowel syndrome (IBS) and seizures. However, if there are too many ketones in the bloodstream this is known as ketoacidosis. If there aren't enough ketones in the blood, that's not ideal either. We are looking for a happy medium; not too high and not too low. This is known as "nutritional ketosis," a term coined by Dr.Stephen Phinney, Chief Medical Officer at Virta Health. It's a safe blood level where ketones can reside to feed the necessary organs of the body. The ketogenic diet allows us to be in a state of nutritional ketosis.

What Exactly is the Ketogenic Diet?

It is a diet that consists of eating low carbohydrate foods, a moderate amount of protein and high amounts of fat. The aim is to replace the carbohydrate intake with fats as this puts your body into a state known as ketosis. Ketosis is a natural metabolic state where the body creates energy by producing ketones using fat instead of carbohydrates. Ketosis occurs when there is a limited amount of blood glucose sugar (the body's preferred fuel for the cells), often during a fast, pregnancy, starvation or during infancy.

To get the body into a state of ketosis it takes 50 grams or less of carbohydrates a day. For this to happen certain foods need to be removed from the diet such as sugary foods and drinks, and grains. Also, you would need to reduce the amount of legumes and fruit you eat. This is why Dr.Lodi discusses that a water fast can help to bring about ketosis within 72 hours, no carbohydrates are being consumed.

In addition to glucose levels dropping during a state of ketosis, hormone insulin levels will also reduce and at this point the fatty acids that are stored in the body's fat will get released. Many of the fatty acids will be transferred to the liver where they are transferred into ketones and can then act as fuel for the body.

This type of diet has been adopted by many cultures throughout history. For example, the Masai in Africa. They have been studied by medical researchers who found that heart disease was very low amidst their population even though their diet mainly consists of fat—saturated fat! Their cholesterol levels were also low. This also applies to the Inuit culture.

Even in the American culture, at one point we were using this diet. For example, Dr.Elliot P Joslin was the first doctor in the USA to specialize in diabetes. He was treating patients who had Type 2 diabetes at a time when insulin injections were not available. He advised his patients (one of them was his mother) to have a low carbohydrate, high fat diet.

There are different types of the ketogenic diet:

1. **Standard ketogenic diet (SKD):** This is a very low carbohydrate, moderate protein, high fat diet. This is the diet Dr.Hallberg

recommends and we will delve deeper into this type of diet in this chapter. In Chapters 8 and 9 we will provide a meal plan and recipes.

2. **Cyclical ketogenic diet (CKD):** This would include a couple of days a week where your diet contains higher carbohydrates and on the other days it's lower.

3. **High protein ketogenic diet:** This is similar to the SKD only you add more protein.

4. **Target ketogenic diet (TKD):** With this diet you would include more carbohydrates around your exercise regime/workouts

With nutritional ketosis or the ketogenic diet, Phinney advises that it's a very powerful tool—when done properly! It isn't just about cutting out carbohydrates. You need to make sure you're receiving important minerals such as sodium, magnesium, zinc, iron, calcium, and potassium (broth, meats, and vegetables). Also, an important point to mention is that for some people with medical conditions it isn't always safe. For example, if you have **high blood pressure and are on medication, you will need to have your doctor supervise you** because at some point the medication will need to be withdrawn as your health conditions start to reverse. If you have **liver disease** or a **heart condition** then careful consideration will need to be given to ensure your safety. Please **be aware** of physicians who are not experienced in doing this. For instance, if you're on certain medications and proceed to start the diet (unsupervised by a doctor), you could reverse the disease which is fantastic, *but,* if you don't take away the medication you could have serious side effects.

This type of diet is so powerful that it is also used to treat the following:

● Epilepsy in children when their medication stops working

● Cancer

● Acne

● Brain injuries

● Polycystic Ovary Syndrome

● Parkinson's disease

● Alzheimer's disease

How the Ketogenic Diet Can Help to Treat Diabetes (Benefits)

First, we must remind you that to be successful on the ketogenic diet, it is important to do it correctly and make sure it is safe. For instance, we advise that you let your doctor know what you are doing. Dr.Phinney advises that if you have **Type 1 diabetes**, you will need special medicalized support. It takes a highly trained physician who knows what they are doing and can closely supervise you, to do this. Someone with **Type 2 diabetes**, it's important that you have a well-trained medical expert who can supervise you, although you won't require as much supervision as something with Type 1 diabetes. The diet:

- Improves endurance

- It's safe (even for growing children)

- Great for most people including athletes

- Decreases triglycerides (bad cholesterol)

- Increases HDLs (good cholesterol)

There's plenty of research that proves a ketogenic diet can treat Type 2 diabetes. For instance, Dr.Hallberg has carried out research on 400 people; 262 have Type 2 diabetes and the remaining 138 have pre-diabetes. The average age of the group is 54 years and the average BMI is 41. Many of the participants have been diagnosed with Type 2 diabetes for many years. The aim of the study was to get the participants to go into nutritional ketosis. They were not on a calorie-restricted diet and in fact, they were advised to eat until they felt full—ensuring that they ate plenty of fat. Their blood ketone levels were frequently checked.

Results of the study

Within 10 weeks of starting the study, the weight decreased by 7.2 percent, on average. Six months later, the weight dropped even further and the average weight loss was 12 percent. Dr.Hallerberg concluded from this study that people who are not restricting calories but are significantly reducing their carbohydrate intake and increasing fats, can lose weight and maintain it over a long period of time.

The trial conducted by Dr.Hallberg also shows that the patients had a huge drop in their blood sugar levels as their A1C levels reduced to 1.0 percent on average. The patients who started the trial on insulin medication, after the first 10 weeks alone a whopping 87 percent of them were able to significantly reduce their medication or eliminate it. The 282 patients who had started with Type 2 diabetes, saw their triglycerides (bad cholesterol) drop by 22 percent!

Further Benefits of the Ketogenic Diet

● There are a lot of misconceptions around nutritional ketosis and the ketogenic diet. Dr.Phinney emphasizes that this type of diet is the most effective in dealing with abdominal fat—the most dangerous type of fat. Dr.Phinney has carried out a study to compare the results of people who take a high carbohydrate, low fat, calorie-restricted diet with people who took a low carbohydrate, high fat diet. After 12 weeks, the people on the low carbohydrate high fat diet lost more weight (around half) than those on the high carbohydrate diet. This includes a greater reduction on abdominal fat.

- People who have pre-diabetes or Type 2 diabetes receive a "prompt response," according to Dr.Phinney in a reduction on blood glucose levels when they start the ketogenic diet. This is because if you are eating less carbohydrates there will be less glucose being produced and so the amount of sugar going into the blood will be reduced. Again, the study showed that there was a significant reduction in blood glucose levels in participants who took the ketogenic diet and no change in those who took the high carbohydrate, low fat diet over a 12-week period.

- It improves insulin insensitivity.

- Dr.Phinney also found that the diet changed the blood lipid values ('good' and 'bad' cholesterols) that can determine if someone gets metabolic syndrome (pre-diabetes). In the study, the people on the ketogenic diet had their 'bad' fats reduce to more than twice the amount of those who were on the high carbohydrate, low fat diet. It's interesting that despite eating more fat on the ketogenic diet, their fat levels still plummeted! These results are greater than what a patient could expect if they were taking medication to control or lower their 'bad' cholesterol levels! These results show that eating animal fats, eggs, and dairy is really not the issue of high 'bad' cholesterol.

The reason many healthcare experts believe it is dangerous to eat saturated fats is because when they measure the blood and it's high in saturated fat it's assumed that the higher the saturated fat in the blood the greater the risk of diabetes, heart disease, cancer, etc. Dr.Phinney argues that people haven't observed the blood with saturated fat once a patient goes into a ketogenic diet. However, Dr.Phinney and others (Hallberg) have, and they noticed blood glucose levels *lowered*. When the body becomes keto-adapted, it's capable of getting rid of saturated fat very easily and so it isn't an issue to consume it. It's all about what your body is able to 'reserve' from what you eat. Saturated fats are not harmful *if* your body is adapted to keto.

● A ketogenic diet trains the body on how to burn fat more effectively. Studies have shown that athletes had more energy on the ketogenic diet than if they were on the low fat, high carbohydrate diet.

- Reduces inflammation in the body.

- With the ketogenic diet, people are able to eat to satiety, according Dr.Phinney and yet within the first 12 weeks of the study, 75 percent of the patients still reduce their body weight.

- General aches and pains diminish.

- Irritable Bowel Syndrome (IBS) goes away.

- Migraine headaches are reduced or go away.

- Amount of fat in the liver goes down.

- Helps the eyes (less risk for cataracts).

- More energy and better sleep.

- Improved memory.

- Feeds the digestive/gut system.

- The body becomes capable of burning almost all of its energy from fat.

Please take into account that Dr.Phinney advises the following:

"...this is a very powerful tool. It can have very beneficial effects on a number of chronic conditions but when a person is taking medicines for those chronic conditions, those beneficial effects usually meant a sharp and rapid reduction on medication and that can be dangerous unless you have the assistance of a physician who understands this type of diet and understands how to manage the medications. This cannot be done in a casual way. You cannot start the diet and then go back and see the physician six weeks later and say, 'so what do you think I should do with my diabetes medication?' because typically we have the most changes in the first six days when people get the diet right."
(Phinney 2018).

Dr.Phinney has also acknowledged that the concern is for a person to find a doctor that understands this. After all, we have already discussed that there is so much conflicting information around when it comes to treating Type 2 diabetes—this is just with the experts who understand it can be treated and 'cured,' let alone the ones who still believe it's incurable! However Dr.Phinney stresses the importance for a person to look carefully when finding a doctor who does understand this as they will need to help them manage the medication in a safe way so that they receive the best results.

Can You Follow the Ketogenic Diet Over the Long-Term?

In short, yes, you can! Dr.Phinney is completely confident that anyone can follow this diet permanently! It's not so much a diet but a new approach and attitude to how we nourish the body. Unlike other diets such as the Mediterranean diet (including low carbohydrate Mediterranean) and the paleo diet, they do not allow for the body to adapt to keto as they either have too much protein or are not sustained enough. The ketogenic diet allows for a healthy balance. For instance, it allows you to keep protein to moderate levels of around 10 to 20 percent and carbohydrates under 10 percent. This means that most of the fuel will be coming from fats. This can be done for years or the rest of your life, not just for weeks or months! It's about cutting out sugary foods, most starchy foods and refined carbohydrates. Instead, you are eating real, whole foods and plenty of delicious foods to satiate your body.

Chapter 8: Meal Plans

The meal plan is based on the ketogenic diet we discussed in the previous chapter. We have chosen to focus on the ketogenic diet not just for its many health benefits but also because it is very flexible. For instance, if you are vegan, lactose intolerant, are a vegetarian or have any other dietary preferences or food restrictions, the ketogenic diet can be adapted to suit your individual needs. You want to enjoy the foods that you consume so if there's anything on the list you really don't like, don't have it. Also, remember to take into consideration any allergies you have. You can use an app to devise a ketogenic diet if you would prefer.

Meal Plan (dos and don'ts)

As a reminder, you want to stay away from the following:

- Grains and starches
- Sugary foods and drinks (including *some* sauces and condiments)
- Alcohol
- Unhealthy oils (vegetable oils)
- Sugar-free foods
- Low-fat, fat-free, and other diet products

- Beans and legumes
- High carb foods and drink

Remember, you want to consume the following:

- Meat
- Oily fish
- Nuts and seeds
- Healthy oils (coconut oil, extra virgin olive oil, avocado oil)
- Eggs
- Avocados
- Condiments (salt, pepper, herbs and spices)
- Unprocessed cheeses (goat)
- Vegetables that are low in carbohydrates (leafy greens, peppers, tomatoes, etc)
- Non-starchy vegetables
- Grass-fed butter and cream

Other Dos

- Remember to consult your doctor or physician first, especially if you have other health conditions and are taking medication.
- Plan ahead with your meals and preparations so that you don't end up snacking on the wrong types of foods.

- Keep your weekly shopping list and meal plan somewhere you can see it, like on the refrigerator so you know where you're up to.

- Try and mix up your recipes rather than sticking to having the same dishes day in and day out, otherwise it's easy to become bored and you may be tempted to fall back into your old routine.

- If you feel hungry in between meals then have a snack—it's okay!

- Drink lots of water or healthy fluids during the first week and ensure your salt levels are adequate.

Menu Sample

	Breakfast	Lunch	Dinner
Monday	Bacon, eggs, sausages, sprinkled with pepper and herbs	Watercress soup	Salmon with green beans or asparagus cooked in garlic butter
Tuesday	Avocado, Egg, Mushrooms and spinach	Chickpea and hazelnut salad	Colorful roasted vegetables
Wednesday	Oatmeal breakfast	Handful of various nuts, celery sticks, carrot sticks, guacamole and salsa dip	Lamb sliders
Thursday	Ginger and spinach Smoothie	Beetroot falafels	Mackerel and egg
Friday	Coconut porridge	Cabbage casserole	Fried cabbage and crispy bacon
Saturday	Mushroom omelette	Chicken Salad	Thai curry cabbage
Sunday	Scrambled or poached egg and avocado	Tofu and veggie wok	Butter fried Broccoli

Desserts/Snacks

- Low-carb ice cream
- Dark chocolate
- Cacao smoothie
- Carob Smoothie
- Fruit salad
- Strawberries and cream
- Nuts and seeds
- Cheese with olives
- Kale chips
- Eggplant fries
- Salad sandwiches
- Onion rings
- Garlic bread
- Sesame crisp bread
- Celery and almond butter

Beverages

- Water

- Unsweetened coffee

- Green tea

- Dandelion tea

- Milk thistle tea

- Sparkling water

- Chicory root coffee

Preparation Tips

- If you don't fancy doing any cooking, you can always take a break from having breakfast and just have some coffee or green tea.

- Why not cook two servings so that you have some for the next day's lunch?

- Why not cook in batches, divide them up into smaller portions, put them in Tupperware and freeze them? You can always warm them up when you're ready to eat them.

- Make a large batch of broth, leave it to cook in the crockpot or slow cooker for 24 to 48 hours (if using beef bones) and then you can store it in the fridge. You can have a warm cup of broth whenever you feel like it.

● Repeat the dishes you love.

● Boil up a batch of eggs and keep them in the fridge as a snack.

● Sardines with some raw vegetables or salad is an easy way to prepare something tasty without having to cook.

Shopping List

Try to keep it as simple as you can. Your shopping list should have the following: Fresh produce, healthy fats and proteins. If you choose fresh *and* frozen produce then you won't have to worry about all of your fresh food going off before you've had a chance to consume them. The following is a guideline to help you. Your shopping list may differ depending on what recipes you choose to cook.

Grass fed Meats: Beef, pork, lamb, venison

Grass fed Poultry: Chicken, duck, turkey

Fish: Wild salmon, mackerel, and sardines

Eggs: Pastured, organic

Dairy: Full fat milk, yogurt, butter, and cream

Dairy free (alternative): Coconut milk, nut milks, soy milk, and coconut cream

Cheese: Unpasteurized goat's cheese, brie, mozzarella, feta, cream cheese, halloumi

Avocados: Organic and whole

Seafood: shrimp, lobster, mussels, oysters

Fresh or frozen vegetables: Cauliflower, broccoli, leafy greens, cabbage, watercress, beets, garlic, onions, green beans, asparagus, mushrooms, zucchini, squashes (various kinds), and sweet potatoes

Fresh or frozen fruits: Strawberries, blueberries, raspberries, and blackberries

Condiments: Salt, pepper, herbs, spices (fresh and dried)

Nuts: Almonds, walnuts, pecans, macadamia, hazelnuts

Nut butters: Peanut butter or almond butter

Seeds: Pumpkin, sesame, flaxseed, chia

Oils: Coconut, avocado, olive oil

Others: Cacao powder, carob powder, dark chocolate (90 - 100%), coconut milk, almond milk, coconut cream, full fat cow's milk, goat's milk, green tea, chicory, dandelion tea, milk thistle, coffee, granola, falafels, coconut flour, tortillas, tofu, chickpeas.

Chapter 9: Recipes

The following recipes are to help give you an idea of dishes you can cook. Remember, it's important that you listen to your body so if there are any ingredients in the recipes that you either don't like or cannot have, then please feel free to either leave out or substitute for something else.

Breakfast Recipes

Bacon, eggs, sausages, sprinkled with pepper and herbs

Serves 1

2 eggs

4 slices of bacon

2 sausages

Fresh parsley (optional)

Salt and pepper (to taste)

Instructions

Using a large pan or wok, fry the sausages over a medium heat for five minutes and then add the bacon. Turn over the sausages occasionally. Cook bacon until crispy and the sausages until they are brown. Set them aside on a plate. Leave the fat in the pan. Next, crack the eggs in the same pan and fry them over a medium heat. Cook eggs however you like them. Add salt and pepper to taste and garnish with parsley. Serve.

Avocado, Egg, Mushrooms and spinach

Serves 1

2 Eggs

1 whole avocado (or half)

¼ cup of mushrooms (chopped)

2 cups of spinach

1 tbsp olive oil

Salt and pepper (to taste)

Instructions

In a medium to large pan, heat one tablespoon of olive oil on medium heat. Then add mushrooms and sauté them for two minutes. Add spinach and remove from pan when starts to wilt. Add a little more olive oil and then cook eggs to however you want them. Serve when ready, add salt and pepper if desired.

Scrambled or poached egg and avocado

Serves 1

1 Egg

½ avocado

A pinch of paprika

Instructions

Chop half an avocado into slices. Place a poached egg or scrambled egg on top and sprinkle with a pinch of paprika.

Mushroom Omelette

Serves 1

3 medium eggs

1 oz of butter (for cooking)

1.oz of grated/shredded cheese

4 large mushrooms or small handful of button mushrooms

¼ chopped yellow onion

Salt and pepper (to taste)

Instructions

Whisk the eggs together in a mixing bowl, using a fork. Add salt and pepper and continue to whisk until frothy. Melt the butter in a frying pan on medium heat, then add the mushrooms and onions. Stir them until soft and add in the egg mixture.

Once the omelette is starting to get firm and cooked, sprinkle the grated cheese on top. Very carefully, fold the omelette in half (ideally, using a spatula). Continue to cook until the omelette is golden brown and then serve on a plate.

Coconut porridge

Serves 1

1 egg

1 oz of butter, coconut butter or oil

3 to 4 tbsp of coconut cream

1 tbsp coconut flour

A pinch of psyllium husk powder

A pinch of salt

Instructions

Beat the egg. Add the coconut flour, psyllium husk powder, salt, and then mix. Melt the coconut cream and butter in a medium-sized pan over a low heat. Slowly, add the egg mixture and combine until you receive a creamy and thick texture. Serve with berries or coconut cream.

Oatmeal breakfast

1 tbsp of whole flax seed (linseed)

1 tbsp of chia seeds

A can of coconut milk or almond milk

1 tbsp of sunflower seeds or sesame seeds

½ tsp of nutmeg or cinnamon (or both)

A pinch of salt

A handful of fresh berries

Instructions

Mix the flax seeds, chia seeds, sunflower/sesame seeds, and coconut/almond milk in a pan and bring to the boil. Reduce the heat and let it simmer. Keep stirring until you have your preferred thick texture— this should only take a minute or two. Turn off the heat. Top with berries, nutmeg, cinnamon and more coconut milk as desired.

Ginger and spinach smoothie

1 tsp of fresh ginger

½ oz of spinach

½ cup of coconut milk, coconut cream or almond milk

¼ tsp juice of lime

¼ cup of water

Instructions

Blend all of the ingredients in a blender until smooth. Serve and enjoy!

Lunch Recipes

Watercress Soup

6 servings

1 cauliflower head

2 garlic cloves

1 white onion

5.3 oz watercress

7.0 oz spinach

4 cups of vegetable, bone or chicken broth

1 cup of coconut cream or milk (plus 6 tbsp to garnish)

¼ cup of coconut oil

Black pepper, parsley and chives to garnish

Instructions

Chop the onion and garlic finely. Heat the coconut oil in a saucepan and then add the onion and garlic. Cook until browned. Cut the cauliflower into small heads and place it in the saucepan with the cooked onion and garlic. Cook for four to five minutes, stirring frequently. Mix in spinach and watercress and cook for two to three minutes. Pour in the stock and bring to boil. Turn the heat down slightly and cook until cauliflower is tender. Next, add the coconut cream or milk and the black pepper and stir gently. Then take the mixture off the heat and use a blender to pulse until smooth and creamy. Serve using parsley and chives to garnish. This can keep in the fridge for up to five days.

Chickpea and hazelnut salad

Serves 2

100g butternut squash, peeled and diced

1 tbsp olive oil

3 oz green beans

1 tbsp hazelnuts

1 tin of chickpeas (drained and rinsed)

8 cherry tomatoes chopped

½ cucumber

a handful of lettuce or your preferred leafy green

½ tsp allspice

2 spring onions, chopped

Instructions

Preheat the oven to 374 degrees Fahrenheit.

Place the butternut squash in boiling water and cover. Let it simmer for five minutes. Take off the boil, drain the water and then place on a baking tray. Pour the olive oil over the butternut squash and then sprinkle the allspice on top. Place the baking tray in the oven and let it cook for 15 minutes until golden brown. Steam the green beans and once cooked set aside. Put the cooked butternut squash in a bowl and add the remaining ingredients, making sure to mix well. Drizzle a little more olive oil on top and then serve.

Beetroot falafels

Makes 10 (falafels)

2 large beets chopped into cubes

2 garlic cloves

A handful of fresh coriander

2 tsps of ground coriander (or dried)

1 tsp of ground cumin

A pinch of salt and pepper

Instructions

Preheat the oven to 392 degrees Fahrenheit. Place the beets on a baking tray and cook for 35 to 40 minutes. When they are cooked, take them out of the oven and set to one side until they are cool *(*you can do this step the night before if you'd prefer)*.

Place all of the ingredients (including the cooked beets) into a food processor and blend until everything has broken down into pieces (not pureed). Next, take small amounts of the broken down mixture, roll into balls and pat them down so they are fairly flat. Place on a broiler and leave to cook for six to eight minutes on a medium/low heat. Alternatively, place in an oven if you'd prefer. Serve with some chilled dip and parsley garnish.

Cabbage casserole

Serves 1

⅓ lbs green or red cabbage (shredded)

¼ oz yellow onion (shredded)

½ oz garlic clove (crushed)

⅔ oz butter or coconut oil

¼ cup of thick whipping cream

1tbsp sour cream

1 oz cream cheese

1/4 tsp of dried parsley

¼ tsp dried chives

A pinch of salt and pepper

1 oz grated/shredded cheese (e.g mozzarella)

Instructions

Preheat oven to 400 degrees Fahrenheit. Heat the butter/coconut oil in a large frying pan. Sauté the cabbage, onion and garlic until softened. Pour in the rest of the ingredients except for the shredded cheese, and simmer for five to 10 minutes. Take off the heat and place in a greased baking dish. Add the shredded cheese and oven cook until the cheese has melted and turned golden (approximately 15 to 20 minutes). Serve.

Chicken salad

Serves 1

1 oz leafy greens chopped

1 oz red and green peppers chopped

1 spring onion chopped

4 cherry tomatoes chopped

4 oz roast chicken

1 tbsp olive oil

Instructions

Mix the vegetables and tomatoes together—toss well. Then add the chicken and pour a tablespoon of olive oil on top. Serve.

Dinner Recipes

Salmon with green beans or asparagus cooked in garlic butter

1 serving

4 oz salmon (in pieces)

4 oz asparagus

1 oz of butter

½ garlic clove

1 tbsp of lemon juice

Instructions

Preheat oven to 400 degrees Fahrenheit. Trim the asparagus. Mince the garlic clove. Place the salmon pieces on foil, on a baking tray along with the asparagus. Rub the minced garlic all over the salmon pieces. Melt the butter on a low heat in a pan. Mix the butter with the lemon juice and pour all over the salmon pieces. Cook the salmon and asparagus for eight to 10 minutes. Serve.

Colorful roasted vegetables

⅙ lb brussel sprouts (outer layer peeled if preferred)

1 ⅓ cherry tomatoes

1 ⅓ mushrooms

A pinch of sea salt and black pepper

½ tsp of dried rosemary or thyme (or a few sprigs fresh).

⅛ cup of olive oil

Instructions

Preheat oven to 400 degrees Fahrenheit. Cut up all the vegetables and place into a baking dish. Add the herbs, salt, pepper, and olive oil. Mix well. Bakes for 20 minutes until cooked. Serve.

Lamb sliders

Serves 1

1 lb ground lamb

¼ tsp of black pepper and salt

½ white or yellow onion diced

¼ garlic clove minced

Small handful of fresh mint leaves chopped

¼ lemon (zest)

Instructions

Preheat grill to medium to high heat. Place the lamb into a bowl and season with salt and pepper, onion, garlic and lemon zest. Mix well. Form six to eight burger patties with the mixture and grill for about four to five minutes on each side or until preferred. Serve on a plate, and garnish with mint leaves.

Mackerel and egg

Serves 1

1 can of mackerel in tomato sauce

2 eggs

1 tbsp of butter or coconut oil

1 oz lettuce or basil (or both)

2 tbsp of olive oil

Salt and pepper to taste

Instructions

Fry the eggs in butter to however you want them. Place the other ingredients on a plate and the eggs. Drizzle with olive oil, sprinkle salt and pepper to taste.

Fried cabbage and crispy bacon

Serves 1

5 oz bacon (chopped into small pieces)

½ lb green cabbage (chopped into small pieces)

1 oz butter

Salt and pepper

Instructions

Fry the bacon in a pan over a medium heat until crispy. Add the cabbage and butter and cook until golden. Add salt and pepper. Serve.

Thai curry cabbage

1/2 tbsp red curry paste

1 1/2 tbsp coconut oil

1/2 tbsp sesame oil

1 lb green cabbage (shredded)

½ tsp salt

Instructions

Heat the coconut oil in a frying pan or wok and then add the curry paste. Stir. Add the cabbage and stir until golden brown. Lower the heat and continue to stir for a minute. Add the salt and sesame seed oil and sauté for two minutes. Serve.

Butter fried broccoli

Serves 1

1 lb broccoli (florets chopped)

3 oz butter

1 scallion (chopped)

Salt and pepper to taste

Instructions

Melt the butter in a pan and sauté the broccoli for four to five minutes until brown and soft. Add the scallion and cook for another two minutes. Add the salt and pepper. Serve with some spicy mayo or any other dip of your choice.

Desserts and Snacks Recipes

Blueberry pancakes

Serves 1

½ cup of almond flour

2 tbsp of coconut flower

½ tsp cinnamon or nutmeg

½ tsp of baking powder

3 eggs

¼ cup of coconut milk, almond milk, goat's milk or cow's milk

¼ cup of fresh or frozen blueberries

Instructions

Add all of the ingredients (except for the blueberries) into a high-powered blender until thick. Then pour the batter into a mixing bowl and stir the berries into the mixture. Leave it to set for five minutes and then add a little more milk if you feel it's too thick. Grease a pan and preheat it (medium to low heat) and then pour small amounts (approximately ¼ cup) of batter at a time and cook for two to three minutes on each side, until golden brown. Once cooked, serve immediately or they can be stored in a fridge/freezer.

Banana waffles

Serves 1

1 peeled banana (ripe)

1 egg

6 tbsp of almond flower

½ tsp of baking powder

⅛ tbsp ground psyllium husk powder

6 tbsp of coconut milk

½ tsp of vanilla extract

⅛ of ground cinnamon

A pinch of salt

Coconut oil for frying

Instructions

Mix or blend all of the ingredients in a bowl until smooth. Using a waffle maker or add coconut oil to a frying pan and then add the mixture.

Serve with some coconut whipped cream or fresh berries.

Full fat yogurt with blueberries and almonds

Serves 1

½ cup of unsweetened full fat greek yoghurt

¼ cup of fresh blueberries

Handful of roasted almonds

Instructions

Dish the yogurt into a bowl, add the blueberries and almonds. Serve and enjoy!

Strawberry Chia Pudding

Serves 4

1 cup of coconut milk

1 cup of almond milk (or milk of your choice)

A small handful of fresh or frozen strawberries

¼ cup of chia seeds

A vanilla bean (optional)

A pinch of salt

A few strawberries for decoration (optional)

Instructions

Blend the coconut milk, almond milk and salt in a blender until well mixed. Add the chia seeds and pulse for for two minutes. Cut open the vanilla bean and scrape the essence into the mixture. Blend again. The chia pudding should start to look thick. Place the mixture into a bowl for up to four hours. This can be made the night before and left in the refrigerator overnight. Serve with strawberries and enjoy!

Cheese Roll-ups

Serves 1

2 oz cheddar cheese or edam cheese in slices

½ oz butter or coconut butter

¼ tsp of drive chives (optional)

Instructions

Lay the cheese slices out on a cutting board. Cut the butter into thin pieces (or use a cheese slicer). Spread the butter onto each cheese slice. Roll up the cheese slices and garnish with dried chives. Serve.

Chapter 10: Listen to Your Heart

In previous chapters we have discussed how the body is an intelligent system that knows what's best for you in every given moment. Unfortunately, due to societal conditioning many of us are not taught to tune in and listen to its messages. Instead, we are encouraged to listen to others about what's right for us. This normally comes at an expense (in more ways than one), our health being the biggest cost. Although we ignore our body's messages, it continues to speak to us, often through discomfort yet we still don't listen. Often, we perceive the messages to be negative, perhaps it's because they can be painful and we want to get rid of the discomfort as soon as possible. For example, when we have a headache, we often take pain relief rather than stop and question why we have a headache in the first place. Also, by relieving the pain with medication it doesn't get to the root cause. The pain may go away temporarily, however the real reason for the health ailment is still present.

The messages we receive from the body in the form of physical conditions may sometimes have something to do with what's going on in our lives. It seems that our bodies and the external environment have a relationship. Whatever is taking place in our external environment we feel the impact, physically, mentally, and emotionally. Actually, when we are experiencing emotions and thoughts it affects our physical health and vice versa. We may not be able to control our external environment completely, but we still need to train ourselves to be more in tune with what's going on with our bodies so that we can make the best choices for our health.

Your Body's Intelligence System

Physician and founder of Santa Cruz Integrative Medicine Clinic, Dr.Rachel Carlton Abrams, has stated: *"R(e)volutionary medicine recognizes that we are not isolated organs systems. Nor are we isolated organisms, but we are part of the environment we live in. We need to take our evolutionary wisdom and add it to the necessary r(e)volution in medicine."* (Abrams 2011).

By listening to the body's messages we are better equipped to deal with health issues or any other situations before they become more difficult.

Dr.Abrams has identified five areas that make up our basic human needs:

1. Eating
2. Moving
3. Sleeping
4. Loving
5. Meaning

Eating

We have evolved to eat small portions of fresh food and not the processed refined foods that contain chemicals.

Moving

We didn't evolve to live a sedentary life. Many of us sit in front of a computer for several hours a day without moving our body—this is not what our ancestors did. Abrams suggests that this is why 80 percent of the population has back pain in the USA alone, while only 10 percent of indigenous cultures have it. She also argues that if we moved more frequently on a daily basis, many of the chronic diseases experienced by most people could be prevented.

Sleeping

We have evolved to sleep in the dark and to get enough until we felt well rested. There was a time when we slept around 10 hours a night. Today, many of us get less than seven hours of sleep, which leads to obesity, depression, poor performance for adults at work and with children at school.

Love

Abrams acknowledges that love is very important for our well-being. She argues that love is essential in helping to keep us healthy and to ward off chronic diseases. We are social creatures. We had to be social, otherwise we wouldn't have survived, and so we have evolved to crave that sense of belonging. She recommends that people connect more with their loved ones.

Meaning

People often like to find meaning in their lives. They want to know that their actions and opinions matter. Dr.Abrams has discussed in her Tedx Talk that what we believe impacts how we feel and the choices and actions we take. She says, *"Having a sense of meaning and purpose in your life, can actually extend your lifespan by years...If we look at the stories of the native peoples of this earth from whom we all originate, they all believed that we are not separate from the earth from which we arise. We co-evolved with the earth over thousands of years. When we get into alignment with our evolutionary nature, not only are we healthier, not only are we happier, but we can heal the diseases of civilization..."* (Abrams 2011).

The mind and body are not separate and although as a society we still view them as being separate, modern day neurologists/neuroscientists have done extensive research only to discover they are deeply interconnected. So, how do we start tuning in to our body's intelligence?

Dr.Abrams has advised that we continue to have our body's checked out fairly regularly so we know how it's doing. Although we can tune in and feel our body there are some things we won't be able to feel, such as our cholesterol (although we may experience symptoms if bad cholesterol is too high). **Measuring** how your body is doing is important. This includes (but not limited to):

1. Your blood pressure
2. Your pulse
3. Your cholesterol

Next, it's important to **sense.** That includes sinking into your body to be able to feel every part of it. It's important to develop this skill. After all, how are you supposed to know when your stomach is full if you can't feel your body? You can't!

So, really **feel** the sensations in your body. Where are the sensations? What do they feel like? It is a stabbing sensation? A pulsation? Does it feel hot? Cold? Heavy? How big does it feel? It may seem a little silly doing this at first but once you get into the habit, it will feel more natural. This is part of being mindful. Be aware that when you feel anxious, nervous, afraid, excited, etc they cause physical sensations in the body so just try to be aware of them. By feeling a sensation, you can then ask yourself what the causation is? For instance, is it associated with memories or anything else?

Discernment is another important factor in this process because it allows you to put all the steps together to determine what your body's message is. As a very general example, someone could be experiencing severe headaches, chest pains, fatigue or an irregular heartbeat quite frequently. They may have their blood **measured** only to find out they have high blood pressure. They will now have a **sense** of what's going on in their body and **feel** the emotions that are connected to the sensations at certain times. For instance, they may notice that they feel the symptoms whenever they are having a conversation with a particular person or even if they are around them. Using their **discernment**, they may come to understand that their blood pressure is high due to their unhealthy relationship with someone. The body could be trying to say, "you need to develop a different relationship with this person". From there, they can start to make different choices that will be more empowering.

Dr.Abrams has emphasized that learning the language of the body is quite a challenging skill, but it can be learned and should be. She also states:

"I often say the sensations are the words—the vocabulary, and the feeling aspect the emotions are the metaphors and discernment is the story." (Abrams).

This process allows us to develop a new relationship with our bodies and the more we have the desire to want to listen to it, the better we'll be able to understand it's messages. Dr.Abrams has acknowledged that 90 percent of illnesses are lifestyle induced. This includes Type 2 diabetes, blood pressure, blood sugar, cholesterol, cancer, etc. They are lifestyle diseases that are caused by what we choose to do and what we are exposed to in our external environment that is out of our control, although many of these can be within our control. Many people do actually know what they should and shouldn't be eating, however they are not listening. There is a reason for this and it could be emotional or psychological. For instance, if you are eating too many sugary foods it could be to do with feeling stressed or due to lack of financial resources, etc. By not listening, you may continue to reach for the sugary snacks or engage in some form of emotional eating as a "pick me up" while continuing with the same stressful situation. It will then have further negative consequences, such as health problems, until you learn to listen to your body and act accordingly. We can rectify this by getting into the habit of listening to our bodies. As mentioned earlier in the book, it's not about blaming and shaming yourself. It's about acknowledging what has occurred and how to change habits. By starting to become aware of them, it's a step in the right direction.

Chapter 11: Live Clean and Pure

Now that we are aware of how we can listen to our bodies, it's time to consider how to create an environment (internally and externally) that will allow for optimum health and well-being. Living a clean and pure life can mean different things to each person. In the context of this guide, it means to live a life that allows you to be the best version of you by surrounding yourself with things that will have you thriving. You can choose to consume fresh and organic foods and clean water. You can also choose to think and believe in a certain way that will have a positive impact on your mental and emotional state. You can also choose (to a certain extent) what you surround yourself with in your external environment.

Healthy Body

The following will help you to build and maintain a healthy body:

- Changing your diet to one that consists of organic, high quality food and drinks that will nourish your body by providing it with everything it needs. Wherever you can, opt for the best quality water you can find. Many people are realizing the importance of drinking higher quality water. Ideally, try and opt for spring water or perhaps filtered water. If you are fortunate enough to live near a spring, all the better as you can fill up bottles of water to take home.

Many plastics are known to contain an industrial chemical called bisphenol A (BPA). It's mainly found in plastic food containers and water bottles and is known to leak out into the food/drink. This is not to scare you but to make you aware. Glass bottles are a good alternative to store drinking water and there are companies these days who are making BPA free plastic bottles and containers.

Since we know that the skin is the largest organ in the body, it's a good idea to try and limit the amount of chemicals and substances you expose your body to. This includes household products as well as cosmetics. Many of these products contain chemicals which are toxic to the system and it means the body has to work even harder to eliminate toxins from your body.

You don't have to suddenly get rid of all of your existing household and beauty products (although you can if you want to). You can always start small. For instance, first take a look at what you use to clean your house. Perhaps you can make a commitment to slowly replace them with products that contain safer ingredients. You can do this gradually, until eventually, your household products have been replaced. You can also do the same with your hair and face products, etc.

● It's important to listen to your body's messages. We have already discussed this and following Dr.Abraham's approach could prove to be beneficial. The aim is to become more aware and perceptive of our body's needs so that we can give it what it wants to keep us healthy and free from pre-diabetes or diabetes.

● We must provide tending loving care (TLC) since it works so hard 24 hours a day, seven days a week to look after us. Book yourself a massage every now and again, or perhaps you can treat yourself to spa days/weekends.

There are many different types of complementary and alternative therapies. For instance, there is aromatherapy, acupuncture, Reiki healing, yoga, and many more. It's a good idea to consider alternative therapies, especially as your body starts to detox from your old lifestyle habits. We would suggest finding one that you feel drawn to and try it.

● It's important to ensure you move your body frequently. As we have already mentioned, you don't need to do vigorous exercise everyday. Just walking more will help enormously. If you can, take the stairs rather than the elevator. Perhaps you could try using an exercise machine while you're watching your favourite television show. Ideally, you want to be able to move about outside, however, doing exercise indoors while watching something is still getting your body moving.

Healthy Mind

● It's important to be mindful of what you are watching and reading. For instance, if you know that when you sit down in the evenings to have your meal and you're feeling distressed by what's being shown on the news, then don't watch it while you are eating (or at all, if it is really impacting you). It comes down to tuning in with the sensations in your body. If we expose our minds to too much negativity, it can cause us to think, feel, and behave in ways that may not be in our best interest. Instead, try to read books that you find funny, inspiring, uplifting, educational and motivational. This also applies to what you choose to watch.

If you are concerned that you don't have enough time to read, you can always listen to audiobooks or podcasts on your commute to work. It will have a much more positive impact on your day if you were to listen to something that will lift your spirits, help improve your mood or is just in alignment with your goals. For instance, you could listen to an audiobook or podcast on tips and advice on reversing Type 2 diabetes or treating pre-diabetes. Doing this helps to train the mind to focus on improving your health. It will motivate you to continue with your exercise regime or healthy eating. You could listen to success stories, especially if you find yourself craving your usual processed food.

● Don't forget to hug! As Dr.Abrahams has emphasized that hugging someone will help to lift your spirits—and theirs! Research has found that when we hug someone it has the following benefits:

1. Reduces stress

2. Improves heart health

3. Reduces your fears

4. Makes you happier

5. May strengthen your immune system

6. Increases your communication with others

7. Hugs are free!

8. There is even a day called National or International Hugging Day!

● Meditation and journaling.

● Goal setting/vision board and affirmations. Many people find that these methods provide results. We have discussed the benefits of writing down your goals, research has proven this can work very well. In addition to writing down your goals, you may want to consider creating a vision board. A vision board is a tool you can use to visualize your goals. It can be an actual board where you stick pictures and words on it that you have cut out from magazines, or sketched yourself. You can get really creative with this. Then once you have your vision board it's important to put it somewhere you can look at it often. It doesn't have to be a board either, it can be a scrapbook, journal or you could make a movie and watch it every morning! So, if it's your goal to lose weight, reverse Type 2 diabetes, get your cholesterol down, become more physically active and eat healthy whole foods. You can find pictures and words that represent these goals and stick them on your vision board.

Affirmations can also be powerful if done correctly. You want to make sure you're saying the affirmation in the present tense, and ideally, it needs to be a positive affirmation rather than focus on the negative. For example, if you have trouble with chronic fatigue and excessive abdominal fat due to insulin resistance, it would be better not to say, "I no longer have chronic fatigue," or "I don't have have a large waist any more." Instead say, "I am vibrant and full of energy" or "I am so grateful that my waist is a healthy size. My body is healthy and balanced." Again, this is an opportunity for you to get creative with what you say. The words you use must feel right for you.

● Laughter is very important and it is known to help strengthen your immune system. Perhaps you could watch more of your favourite comedies and a little less of the movies, shows or news that leave you feeling depressed, fearful or anxious.

Healthy (External) Environment

There is a saying, "You are who you hang around with." If you spend most of your time with people who complain a lot and see the glass as being half empty, chances are you may pick up on some of their habits or you may be left feeling gloomy after being in their presence. It doesn't mean you should completely cut these people out of your life if you don't want to or feel that you can't, but it may benefit you to cut down on the amount of time you spend with them. Perhaps as you move further along on your healthy lifestyle journey, you may find yourself naturally wanting to seek out people or groups that are more in alignment with your goals and new vision.

If weight loss and better health is a main goal for you and you have a group of friends who have an unhealthy lifestyle and don't want to change it, you may find it becomes increasingly difficult for you to spend so much time with them. If you feel their bad habits (which used to be yours) negatively influence you then it may be time for you to walk away completely. There's no ultimate 'right' or 'wrong' choice, only what feels right for you.

To help encourage yourself to be in an environment that is clean and pure, consider the following:

- Spend time in nature. This can include in mountains, woods, the desert, forrest, or by the sea.

- Re-decorate your home if you are not happy with the interior. Choose colors that give you a sense of well-being. Think about what you are looking for. Do you want more calmness and peace in your life? Are you looking to be more vibrant and energetic? Colors affect our moods so it's best to first think about how you want to feel most of the time and then choose your colors accordingly.

- If re-decorating your home is not financially viable for you right now, then perhaps you could add a few things around the home. For example, a little water feature or even a bowl of water, if you find that water helps to balance you. You could light some candles, or have a picture of loved ones on your bedroom wall so that you see it first thing in the morning. You could stick positive affirmations around the house and on your refrigerator door. You can just stick up words like, 'healthy,' 'strong,' and 'peaceful.' It may be a good idea for your to have things around the home that represent the four elements: air, water, earth and fire. So, for air, you could make sure you keep the windows open on a daily basis so that clean fresh air can enter and circulate the house. For earth, you may want to have some plants and flowers around the home.

- Music. Maybe you could have relaxing music on in the background—if relaxation, peace and calmness is what you are looking for.

- Don't neglect your workspace environment either. Perhaps you could have a small plant at your desk or a screensaver that shows a place that lifts your spirits whenever you look at it. You could even take a photo of your vision board and use that as your screensaver. Why not have a photo or two of your loved ones on your desk?

There are many things you can do to help improve your environment and they can be inexpensive. You may want to make big changes to your environment straight away, or you may choose to make small improvements every so often. It's your life and your choice!

Conclusion

Type 2 diabetes is an epidemic (some healthcare experts say it's a pandemic) with over 100 million people in the USA alone living with either prediabetes or Type 2 diabetes and many of them haven't yet been diagnosed. It's predicted to increase significantly by 2030. Not only does having prediabetes or Type 2 diabetes cause further problems with health, it's also costing the economy a great deal of money in terms of medical expenses. Despite the alarming rate in which this condition is negatively impacting most of the populace, research has shown it can be rectified.

There are numerous studies that prove prediabetes and Type 2 diabetes can be reversed when someone undertakes major lifestyle changes. This includes changing the diet, exercising and managing stress.

Prediabetes is the condition that occurs before diabetes. When someone has prediabetes it means there blood glucose sugar levels are high in the blood but not high enough to be considered diabetes. Type 2 diabetes occurs when the pancreas is unable to produce enough insulin, or the cells are not reacting properly to the insulin that's being produced. This affects the blood glucose from being able to enter the cells to provide energy. Instead, glucose builds up in the blood. Type 1 diabetes is when the body is unable to produce insulin at all. It is currently not considered

149

to be 'curable.' However, in this ebook we have discussed how prediabetes and Type 2 diabetes is curable and it's a matter of changing your mindset to help prepare you for a healthier lifestyle change that's sustainable over the long haul.

Prediabetes doesn't have any obvious symptoms but you are more likely to have it if you are overweight, live a sedentary lifestyle or have high blood pressure and high cholesterol. This applies to having a higher amount of 'bad' fats and lower levels of 'good' fats. For mothers who have given birth to a baby who weighed more than nine pounds at birth, they too are at risk. Also, if you have a close family member who has Type 2 diabetes you are also considered to be at a higher risk. With Type 2 diabetes, there are some symptoms you may experience:

- Always feeling thirsty.

- Needing to urinate more.

- Feeling tired all the time.

- Blurred vision.

If you suspect you may have prediabetes or Type 2 diabetes then please do arrange to have the necessary tests. There are three main tests that can be carried out to check if you have prediabetes or diabetes. One of them is an A1C test which measures the average blood glucose sugar levels over a two to three month period. So, even if the test shows you have normal blood sugar levels overall, you may still have high fasting blood sugar. If your test does show that you have normal blood sugar levels, it doesn't mean you may not have Type 2 diabetes. This type of test is used to diagnose prediabetes or diabetes because it doesn't require people to fast beforehand so the tests can be taken at anytime. It's important to understand your diagnosis. When you are diagnosed with a condition like diabetes it isn't the end of the world.

There's the idea that when you have a disease or illness you need to "fight" it off. When we hear about someone (or ourselves) having contracted a disease, there is often a sense of panic and thoughts may be rushing through our heads: "Is this curable?" "Are we going to die?" "How could this have happened?" "How will this affect my life?" It doesn't help that when people are diagnosed, a medical professional's approach can often seem quite frightening or intimidating. For instance, they may tell the patient that although there's nothing that can be done to reverse the disease and that making some changes to their lifestyle such as diet and exercise may help, taking medication for the rest of their lives is the only way to manage symptoms if the disease is considered 'manageable'.

Remember, you don't have to rely on drugs to manage your diabetes, there are other ways and we have taken a look at how you can really start to shift your mindset with the disease. When someone has pre-diabetes it doesn't mean that Type 2 diabetes is inevitable.

The more you educate yourself on your condition the chances are your desire to make changes will deepen.

In chapter three, we learned some tips on how to reduce insulin resistance. It has been estimated that around 80% of people who are overweight are also living with Type 2 diabetes. If a person has a body mass (BMI) that is over 30, they are at a higher risk. It is accepted that being obese actually imbalances the body's metabolism, which in turn causes fat tissue (adipose tissue) to release fat molecules into the bloodstream. This then impacts the insulin responsive cells making insulin less sensitive. Symptoms include having a large abdominal, high blood pressure and high blood sugar.

Three ways you can start to reduce insulin resistance is by adopting the right mindset, changing your habits and behaviors and taking action to maintain a healthy lifestyle.

There are certain foods that must be eliminated immediately. Although there a number of healthcare experts that have different opinions as to what diet should be adopted, in general, most agree that the following foods should be eliminated or reduced:

- White bread

- White pasta

- White rice

- Food and drinks that are high in sugar or salt

- High glycemic foods including melons, pears, apples, pineapples

- Some fruit and dried fruit. Although there are some studies that suggest blueberries, pears and apples are good at helping to prevent diabetes.

- Foods that contain the following ingredients: Glucose, dextrose, glucose syrup, sugar, icing sugar, and sucrose.

- Fries

- Savoury snacks

- Jam, honey, marmalade.

- Limit alcohol intake.

- In a nutshell, all refined foods!

- Stop smoking.

The following foods are known to help reverse pre-diabetes and Type 2 diabetes:

- Leafy greens including kale, spinach, watercress, chard, cabbage, collard, lettuce, and broccoli.

- Beets. Like most vegetables, beets are high in antioxidants and contain phytochemicals that are known to stabilize blood glucose and insulin levels. Beets cleanse the blood and help to reduce insulin resistance.

- Other cruciferous vegetables such as cauliflower, Brussels sprouts, turnips, and radishes.

- Other non-starchy vegetables such as onions, garlic, peppers, mushrooms, asparagus, green beans, cucumber, eggplant, zucchini, and squash.

- Fresh and dried herbs: Parsley, basil, cinnamon, dill, cumin, ginger, rosemary and dandelion.

- Citrus fruits including grapefruit, oranges, lemons, and limes.

- Avocado

- Tomato (they are fruit not a vegetable).

- Chia seeds
- Walnuts
- Almonds
- Pumpkin seeds
- Oats
- Barley
- Quinoa
- Flax seeds
- Brazil nuts
- Hemp seeds
- Cashew nuts
- Amaranth
- Millet
- Sardines
- Salmon, mackerel, herring, trout, pilchards, and fresh tuna.

Keeping the body active is important but it doesn't have to include exercise that you find strenuous. You may decide to take a brisk walk once or twice a day. If you decide to plan an exercise regime, try and think of exercises you can carry out inside the home and ones you can do outside, that way you have options depending on the weather—so you can't let excuses get the better of you. For example, if it's raining heavily on a morning that you had intended to go jogging, rather than tell yourself you can't exercise because of the weather (some people still jog in the rain), you can instead take up the indoor exercise you have as a back-up plan.

Dr.Hallberg has carried out a number of studies and experiments, as have other researchers and they have concluded that reducing carbohydrates, consuming moderate amounts of protein and increasing fat intake will reverse Type 2 diabetes in a short amount of time. Some experts believe that a low-fat plant-based diet is the best way to go while others like Hallberg believe a high fat, low-carbohydrate is effective.

This ebook has intended to provide you with a deeper understanding of what diabetes and pre-diabetes are and how they can be treated. We have looked into how they can be reversed naturally which has been proven by various clinical trials over the years. We have also explored different methods and strategies you can start to do to help you change your lifestyle. For instance, we discussed how mindset techniques such as meditation, goal setting and being mindful in every moment can help you to align your mind and body for optimum healing.

We have also mentioned the importance of listening to your body's intelligence and how you can start to do that. When you make a conscious effort to listen and act according to what your body wants you will find that your health and other areas of your life begin to improve. When you meditate or journal you are better able to gain insights into experiences and situations that you may not have received had you not engaged in either of these practices. Meditation and journaling will also help to increase your intuition and help you tune into your body's needs.

This guide also provides you with a few options on a diet you may find suitable to help you reverse your condition. If you prefer to stick to vegan or raw vegan then Dr.Barnard or Dr.Lodi's suggestions may resonate with you. However, if you want to continue to eat many foods you like then Dr.Hallberg's approach may be better suited to your needs. You can always try one diet and over time, if you don't feel it is right for you then change it to another. Remember, you know better than anyone what your body needs, it's just a matter of tuning into it. Even if you believe you have never before listened to your body and are convinced you don't know how to, *you can*. Just start taking action today and you will be surprised! However, for your safety, we do advise that you find a well-trained physician who can supervise your new diet plan, especially if you take medication for other health conditions.

We wish you all the best on your journey to health and happiness and know that if you apply the steps that have been discussed in this book, your life will improve significantly.

The end... almost!

Reviews are not easy to come by.

As an independent author with a tiny marketing budget, I rely on readers, like you, to leave a short review on Amazon.

Even if it's just a sentence or two!

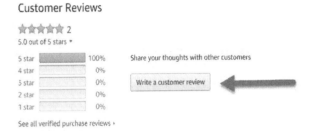

So if you liked the book, please leave a review.

I am very appreciative for your review as it truly makes a difference.

Thank you from the bottom of my heart for purchasing this book and reading it to the end.

Further Resources

Barnard N., *Tackling diabetes with a bold new dietary approach*. (2012). TEDxFremont
https://www.youtube.com/watch?v=ktQzM2IA-qU

Fung J, MD. https://www.dietdoctor.com

Hallbert S., *Reversing Type 2 diabetes starts with ignoring the guidelines*. (2015). TEDxPurdueU
https://www.youtube.com/watch?v=da1vvigy5tQ

Leslie WS., Sattar N., McCombie L., Barnes A., Kennon B., Taylor R & Lean MEJ. *The Diabetes Remission Clinical Trial (DiRECT): protocol for a cluster randomised trial*. (2016). BMC Family Practice.

Lodi T. *How to Get Rid of Diabetes*. (2015).
https://www.youtube.com/watch?v=98MXvH9jxVQ

Lodi T (MD). *Learn How To Reverse Diabetes*. (2016).
https://drthomaslodi.com/how-to-reverse-diabetes

Mikus CR., Oberlin DJ., Libla JL, Taylor AM., Booth FW & Thyfault JP. *Lowering Physical Activity Impairs Glycemic Control in Healthy Volunteers*. (2012). Medicine & Science in Sports & Exercise: February 2012 - Volume 44 - Issue 2 - p 225–231.

National Institute of Diabetes and Digestive and Kidney Diseases (NIDDK). https://www.niddk.nih.gov/

Phinney S,. *Dr. Stephen Phinney on the Safety and Benefits of a Ketogenic Diet (Part 2)*. (2018). Virta Health.
https://www.youtube.com/watch?v=CHJmqhMzKtE

Physicians Committee For Responsible Medicine. *Diet and Diabetes: Recipes for Success.* (N.D).
https://p.widencdn.net/smvqjo/Diet-and-Diabetes-Recipes-for-Success

(R)evolutionary Medicine: Rachel Abrams at TEDxSantaCruz
https://www.youtube.com/watch?v=vUP0yt-6ba4

https://www.diabetes.co.uk/high-intensity-interval-training.html

Rowley WR (MD)., Bezold C, (PhD)., Arikan Y (BA)., Byrne E (MPH)., & Krohe S (MPH). *Diabetes 2030: Insights from Yesterday, Today, and Future Trend.* (2017). Population Health Management.

Trapp, EG., Chisholm, DJ., Freund J., & Boutcher SH. *The effects of high-intensity intermittent exercise training on fat loss and fasting insulin levels of young women.* (2008). *International Journal of Obesity* volume 32, pages 684–691.

Yancy WS., Foy M., Chalecki AM., MC., & Westman EC. Low-*Carbohydrate, Ketogenic Diet to Treat Type 2 Diabetes.* (2005). Nutr Metab (Lond). 2005; 2: 34.
https://www.ncbi.nlm.nih.gov/pmc/articles/PMC1325029

https://www.self.com/story/what-is-high-intensity-interval-training-benefits

https://www.virtahealth.com

Made in the USA
Middletown, DE
01 February 2020